Overcoming Common Problems

Living with Birthmarks and Blemishes

GORDON LAMONT

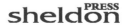

First published in Great Britain in 2008

Sheldon Press
36 Causton Street
London SW1P 4ST

Copyright © Gordon Lamont 2008

The author and publisher have made every effort to ensure that the
external website and email addresses included in this book are correct and
up to date at the time of going to press. The author and publisher are not
responsible for the content, quality or continuing accessibility of the sites.

British Library Cataloguing-in-Publication Data
A catalogue record for this book is available from the British Library

ISBN 978-1-84709-009-6

1 3 5 7 9 10 8 6 4 2

Typeset by Fakenham Photosetting Ltd, Fakenham, Norfolk
Printed in Great Britain by Ashford Colour Press

Produced on paper from sustainable forests

Living with Birthmarks

Gordon Lamont is a radio producer, writer, ⎯ ⎯ ⎯ ⎯ ⎯ ⎯ .ei. His previous books include *The Confidence Book* (Sheldon⎯ ⎯ ⎯ ⎯ 2007), *The Creative Teacher*, with Rosemary Hill (Arts Council, 2005), *The Creative Path* (Azure, 2004) and *Work–Life Balance*, with Ronni Lamont (Sheldon Press, 2001). The author's Confidence Site at <www.theconfidencesite.co.uk> offers confidence tips and techniques, and has much information of relevance to readers of this book including links to all the websites mentioned in the text.

Overcoming Common Problems Series

Selected titles

A full list of titles is available from Sheldon Press,
36 Causton Street, London SW1P 4ST and on our website at
www.sheldonpress.co.uk

Overcoming Common Problems Series

Overcoming Common Problems Series

Contents

Acknowledgements

The author would like to thank the many individuals who have shared their personal stories for this book. Thanks also go to Dr Tom Smith, who kindly read the medical sections of the book.

Introduction

Then I put my hair aside, and looked at the reflection in the mirror, encouraged by seeing how placidly it looked at me. I was very much changed – O very much.

Esther, Chapter 36, *Bleak House*, Charles Dickens

Are you, like Esther and many of the people you will meet in this book, someone whose face stands out because of some unusual feature, such as a birthmark or other facial mark? How do you live with this, how does it affect you in life, in love, in your career and in social situations? Are there negative aspects to it that you would like to change?

Are you a parent of a child with some kind of distinctive facial feature? Do you worry about how you can help your child?

Are you involved in the worlds of medicine or social work or therapy? What issues do you need to be aware of and how can you best advise your clients and patients if they come to you with concerns about a facial abnormality?

A birthmark, blemish or distinguishing mark of any kind may be an ongoing source of distress, often felt much more keenly than others might realize. Even relatively minor markings may make life a misery for those who have them, causing self-consciousness and lack of confidence – even when, as is often the case, other people do not really notice them. This can apply not only to the person with a significant birthmark, such as a port wine stain (like me), but also to a wide range of skin conditions, including disorders of the veins, facial redness and acne. Those with other skin conditions that are visible, such as burns and scars, including acne scars, and conditions resulting in skin discolouration, such as vitiligo, will also experience such feelings.

Interestingly, it has been my experience that others honestly do not seem to notice whether I cover my birthmark (on the left side of my face) with make-up or not. If I do, they often cannot put their finger on what is different. They tend to make remarks such as, 'You look well – been on holiday?'

The point is, how I feel about it and how the outside world sees it are often very different. Of course, I am not naïve enough to think that no one ever notices my birthmark or wonders about that different-looking patch of skin, but I do know that many do not notice it at all and, for those who do, the effect is far less marked and more fleeting than I think it is.

This book explores these and other related issues. I have brought together the experiences of a number of people who have lived with birthmarks and other facial marks and, as well as giving resources for getting help and advice, I talk about how to live with your face and love it.

The Vascular Birthmarks Foundation Europe notes on its website (http://vbfeurope.org) that some 40,000 children are born every year in the United States with a birthmark, of which 85 per cent are on the head or neck. Of children born in the UK, 1 in 10 has some kind of birthmark, but 70 per cent of these disappear naturally over time if left alone (Denise Winterman, 'In your face', online BBC News Magazine, 21 July 2006, available at <http://news.bbc.co.uk/1/hi/magazine/5194394.stm>). Clearly this is a health issue that affects many people across the world. This book, therefore, aims to help all those whose confidence is affected because of some kind of facial abnormality or their perception of it (as well as their carers). There is information on treatments as well, but there is not sufficient space here to explore all the options for all conditions, so the focus is mainly on birthmarks and similar facial features. I have also had to restrict myself to 'minor' blemishes and marks rather than facial disfigurement of a more radical kind, such as that following surgery for facial cancer or a car accident or severe burns. Falklands veteran and inspirational speaker Simon Weston OBE comes to mind in this context. Simon, a Welsh Guardsman, suffered serious facial burns when his ship the Sir Galahad was bombed. His positive approach to getting on with his life continues to be an inspiration to many. Much of the information, many of the stories and some of the ideas in this book will be useful to those with more serious conditions of this kind, but, for more targeted information, get in touch with The Face Trust, of which Simon Weston is patron (visit <www.thefacetrust.org>), and Changing Faces (visit <www.changing faces.org.uk>).

The book is divided into the following chapters:

1 Birthmarks and skin conditions
This chapter discusses various marks, their causes and treatment options.

2 Acne
Acne is a very common problem, affecting not just adolescents but adults as well. It can carry a substantial risk of scarring. This chapter looks at how to treat acne so as to prevent scarring as far as possible.

3 Like your look
Collected here are the stories of people who have chosen not to attempt to hide or seek treatment for their facial marks or have stopped treatment at a certain point and are now proud to show their true face to the world. I hope that they will be inspirational and will help you to consider your own treatment options in a rounded, informed manner.

4 Camouflage
In this chapter I take a look at camouflage cream or make-up, its appropriateness, where to get it and how to use it, with advice and stories from male and female perspectives.

5 Laser treatment
What are lasers and what do they do? This chapter covers the advantages and disadvantages of opting for this treatment, and personal stories from those who have had it and those who have chosen not to.

6 Confidence
Does your mark drain you of your self-confidence? Here are some tips and strategies for facing the world more confidently.

7 Advice for parents
This chapter looks at how to deal with your initial reactions and what help is available. It also covers the subject of how and when to talk to your child about his or her mark.

Being different

As a young child, I knew that it was there. There is a difference, though, between knowing something as a child and knowing it as an adolescent, just as there is another kind of knowing in adulthood and, I am now discovering, something different again in and after the midlife transition.

It really hit me as I entered adolescence, around the time I went to secondary school. Everything hits us at that age.

As adults we can talk and write blithely about 'maelstroms of emotions' or 'churning angst', 'uncertainty', 'confusion' and so on and we tend to see adolescence as a stage we go through, a transition – we see it in perspective. I suspect that we do this as a safety mechanism. Just as my friend Peter has this theory that no one can truly communicate the difficulties of rearing your children because, if they did, the race would die out and, just as it is said that mothers fail to remember the true experience of childbirth because to do so would result in a world of one-child families, so I think that if we could fully recall the experience of adolescence and carry it with us through our lives, we'd find it hard to function as adults. Make no mistake, adolescent angst is real and, although we may think that life is tougher as an adult, this may just be our coping mechanism.

So, at secondary school, my birthmark moved from being a fact to being a factor. It changed from being a thing to being the thing in relation to my confidence. Up until that time, I do not remember any of my contemporaries commenting on it, I do not remember anyone nicknaming me because of it (that does not mean they didn't, just that their comments did not 'stick', did not bother me much). However, then, my 'friends' started to call me 'Blotch' or 'Belisha Beacon', which, for those of you who do not know, were orange flashing lights to mark a safe road crossing named after the Minister of Transport who introduced them in 1934. Now there's a legacy! As a result, I suddenly believed that I had this glowing signal on my left temple, defining me for all to see so that they could mock me.

Children can be cruel and, when that cruelty gains momentum from the power surge of adolescence and the group-think of the mob without the braking perspective of adulthood, some genuine nastiness can ensue. Here is an example. I did some of my classes with Alan – a boy with a very severe case of acne. His face was a mass of red spots and he frequently went to hospital for treatments, but they did not seem to make any difference. At the time when I was being mocked for my birthmark, I was joining in the most unpleasant mocking of Alan. I remember one incident in a geography class when three of us rolled up our books to make 'telescopes' and, looking at Alan, we pretended to be looking at the cratered surface of the moon and we made sure that Alan heard us. You would think that I would be likely to be sensitive to Alan's condition, but humans in groups do not work like that. The odd one out is often only too pleased to unite with his tormentors in picking on a new target and, for adolescents, this is doubly so as there is a strong need then to join in, be one of the gang.

This book is partly about those things that make us different, make us stand out, which is something many people have to live with – the one person in a group with a stammer or a different sexuality or a different racial background than the others. The difficulties people face in all these situations have some common threads running through them: they result from ignorance, prejudice; overcoming them calls for having pride in yourself, coping strategies and so on. However, in this book, I focus on those unique factors that are to do with our faces.

The face we present

To everyone else, our faces are 'us' to a large extent. Think of your favourite teacher. What do you see? His or her face. Perhaps you do not see only the person's face, but it will certainly be the main part of the image that comes into your mind.

I think of a wonderful and inspiring teacher from my early years in secondary school. I see his features, by which I mean his facial features, and, although they are attached to an image of his body, it could be interchanged with those of several other people. What makes him 'him' to me is his face. I suspect that you find the same with the image you have of the person you are thinking of. There are exceptions of course, particularly if the person you have in mind has a very attractive body.

You only have to think of the number of common phrases that use the word 'face' – 'face it', 'face the future', 'face-off' and so on – to know that our faces are important; they are a large part of our definition of self. They exclusively carry the organs responsible for four of the five senses – sight, sound, taste and smell – and the lips have a powerful role in the fifth, touch. Biologists are now adding other senses, such as our internal clock and our sense that our bladder is full, but, in terms of the traditional senses that interface with the world, we experience people and our environment mostly through our faces and other people experience us in largely the same way.

Perfect faces?

There are all kinds of ideas about what makes the perfect face. I take them all with a pinch of salt because, in the end, this is a subjective matter. Did Charlie Chaplin have the ideal face? Well, he had the ideal face for being Charlie Chaplin.

The scientific research on this subject is based on reactions and statistics – the majority of people find this or that attractive. In subjective areas such as this, however, you might choose to be the odd one out and a majority decision means nothing if the face you find most attractive ticks none of these supposedly 'ideal' boxes.

That caveat out of the way, there seems to be some consensus about the importance of symmetry, with many studies suggesting that men in particular have a preference for a symmetrical face in a life partner. It is argued that asymmetry might suggest underlying genetic problems, so we have evolved a love of symmetry ('What makes you fancy someone?', in 'The Science of Love', Science & Nature: Hot Topics, BBC.co.uk, 18 November 2004, p. 3, available online at <www.bbc.co.uk/ science/hottopics/love/attraction.shtml>). My face is somewhat asymmetrical, but I think that makes it interesting! My children are bright and able so the theory has not applied in my case, although my wife's genes could have something to do with that!

Given that our faces are so central to our sense of self and how others interact with us, just how important are those supposedly crucial first impressions? Again, research has been carried out on this question and again I am a little sceptical about the results.

In the worlds of training and business, the 'seven second' theory is often mentioned. For example, business guru Roger Aisles says 'seven seconds is all that people need to start making up their minds about you' (Roger Aisles, 'Your first seven seconds', *Fast Company*, 15 May 1998, p. 184, available online at <www.fastcompany.com/online/15/firstseconds.html>). Search the Internet and books and you will find endless references to this magic figure of seven seconds, but I have not been able to verify that the claims for it have been proven conclusively. In fact, I am not sure how you could and why you would want to.

This said, it is generally agreed that first impressions count and our facial features are an important factor in that. What is less clear is how important those early impressions are overall and to what extent they form a barrier to revised opinions.

Our actions and reactions

Facial identity is a complicated area, but our sense of self, related to our ideas of what we look like, can be strongly tied to our emotional reactions. Even though this relationship between face, our internal image of ourselves, our emotions and our confidence is undoubtedly complex, I am clear on one thing: we can learn to take responsibility for not just our actions but also our reactions. How others respond to us is their affair; how we respond should be our concern. Indeed, that is the essential reason for writing this book.

If you are concerned in any way about facial marks – either your own, a loved one's or even your reaction to the marks of others – that concern can lead to action. That might be in the form of medical intervention, wearing camouflage cream or changing your hairstyle, but could also be to gain perspective on your situation by listening to the stories of others and understanding what you are thinking and feeling. This can lead to changes in our views regarding ourselves and others.

My hope is that this book will offer you some options for change and, through it, you will move forward to face the world in a more positive way.

1

Birthmarks and skin conditions

This chapter offers a brief description of some of the commonest facial marks and treatments for them. It is not an exhaustive list, so I strongly recommend that you have a discussion with your doctor about any facial mark and, if necessary, obtain a referral to the appropriate specialist. Then, even if you opt not to have any treatment, you will know what the mark is and what treatments are available. This is especially recommended for parents and carers of children and babies, as early intervention can, in many cases, completely remove facial marks in the very young or you could be reassured that they are likely to disappear naturally.

In addition to birthmarks, a variety of other conditions can affect the skin. Some problems may be part of another condition that affects other parts of the body, such as lupus, while others affect the skin only and relate to problems with blood vessels, such as varicose veins, or pigmentation or colouring, such as vitiligo. Acne is a common cause of misery in adolescents and can persist beyond the teenage years – this is the case for 1 in 20 adults. Scarring is another issue, which may be the result of an accident, burns or acne. It is also worth remembering that each year more than three million operations are carried out in the UK, many of which leave some form of scarring.

Birthmarks

Birthmarks are called 'voglie' in Italian and 'wiham' in Arabic, meaning 'wishes', underlining the fact that popular mythology has long held birthmarks to be related to events during pregnancy – unsatisfied wishes or cravings, stress or trauma. This just isn't so. There is always an underlying physical cause, even if it is not known exactly why such marks develop.

There are several different types of birthmarks, but, broadly, they can be divided into vascular and pigmented birthmarks. Vascular ones are those that are caused by the blood vessels in the skin, while pigmented are caused by the skin's pigment – the substance that gives colour to the skin (as well as eyes and hair). Also, although they are called 'birthmarks', some may not show up for a few weeks after a baby's birth.

Vascular birthmarks

These marks are formed by abnormal blood vessels in the skin. There are many different types of this kind of birthmark, but the three main ones are:

- salmon patches, or, naevus simplex
- strawberry marks, or, infantile haemangiomas
- port wine stains, or, naevus flammeus.

Strictly speaking, only salmon patches and port wine stains are birthmarks as strawberry marks usually appear in the first few weeks after a baby has been born rather than being present from birth.

Salmon patches

These are the commonest of the vascular birthmarks, occurring in around a third to one half of newborns. They are present at birth as flat, dull red or pinkish areas on the eyelids or forehead (where they may be called an 'angel's kiss'), bridge of the nose, the upper lip and on the nape of the neck (where they are sometimes referred to as 'stork bites').

Usually inconspicuous, they are more noticeable when the child is crying, when they tend to become darker. Most of them fade during infancy, though 50 per cent of those on the nape of the neck persist into adult life. As they are usually covered by hair, they cannot be seen and no treatment is needed.

Strawberry marks

These are soft, raised swellings on the skin, often with a bright red surface, hence the name. They are also known as 'strawberry naevi' or 'infantile haemangiomas'. They appear after birth, usually in the first month, and can occur anywhere on the skin. They are more of a problem when they affect the face or nappy area.

While the cause of strawberry marks is not fully understood, they are a benign overgrowth of blood vessels in the skin, made up of cells that usually form the inner lining of blood vessels. Strawberry marks affect up to 1 in 10 newborn white babies, according to the British Association of Dermatologists and the British Skin Foundation, but are much rarer in Asian and black babies – around 1 in 100. Many of the marks are quite minor and it is these that are very common. Strawberry marks are particularly common in premature babies.

These marks tend to start small and then to grow, most reaching their final size in three to nine months. They then start to fade, quite slowly. Around a third disappear by the age of three and most by school age.

Usually there is only one strawberry mark, but sometimes several come up at the same time. They can appear on any area of skin, but most tend to be on the face and neck. If the haemangioma is within the skin, it will be bright red, like a strawberry, but, if it is located a little deeper, it may appear blue.

While the vast majority of strawberry marks need no treatment, a few do need early attention if they are near strategic areas, such as the eyes, nose or mouth, and their growth threatens to interfere with vision, breathing, feeding and passing urine or stools. They may also need to be treated if they grow very rapidly.

An example of when a strawberry mark would require treatment is Kasabach-Merritt syndrome. This is an extremely rare disorder in which a haemangioma grows to become a reddish-brown tumour. Such a tumour is usually found on the surface of the skin and is sometimes associated with problems with blood clotting.

Children with more than three strawberry marks may need to have a scan to check if there are any internal haemangiomas as these can lead to problems if they go undetected and untreated. The two main forms of treatment are laser and steroids.

Bleeding Sometimes strawberry marks, like other skin, may bleed if bumped or scratched. As with any such injury, the area should be cleaned with soap and water and firm pressure applied with a gauze bandage or cotton wool. If the bleeding does not stop, consult your doctor. You should do the same in the case of itching or infection.

Laser treatment and strawberry marks

Laser treatment has no long-term impact on the outcome of most strawberry birthmarks, research suggests. Dr Kapila Batta of the Birmingham Children's Hospital NHS Trust and colleagues found that many children with strawberry birthmarks appear to do just as well when doctors let the mark disappear naturally as when laser therapy is used (K. Batta, et al., 'Randomized controlled study of early pulsed dye laser treatment of uncomplicated childhood haemangiomas: Results of 1-year analysis', *The Lancet*, 17 August 2002, 360, pp. 521–7). They found that the birthmarks were as likely to disappear by the time children were one year old if they were left alone as they were after laser therapy. The researchers compared treatment with lasers to no treatment in babies from 1 to 14 weeks old who had early, uncomplicated strawberry birthmarks. They excluded children with large facial lesions, those with mixed and deep types of haemangiomas and those involving the eyelid from the study.

Port wine stains

Port wine stains are red or purple marks on the skin. They are usually present at birth, when they may be deep pink, and darken as the baby grows. Port wine stains occur in about 3 out of every 1000 births.

It is thought that these birthmarks form in areas lacking the small nerves that control the ability of blood vessels to constrict. As a result, the blood vessels stay open all the time, which shows up as a permanent blush in the area. Unlike strawberry marks, port wine stains do not fade with time and, in adulthood, they may become thicker and bumpy, bleeding easily if scratched.

Treatment   Laser treatment, using pulsed dye lasers, helps most people, particularly if the mark is on the face, but may not clear the port wine stain completely. Depending on the size and site of the birthmark, up to ten treatment sessions may be required at intervals of eight weeks or so, usually under anaesthetic.

Port wine stains on the limbs respond less well than those on the face. Treatment given early in life, before the birthmark thickens, is more successful than when it is given later on.

Cosmetic camouflage of these marks is often very helpful (see Chapter 4).

Most port wine stains are harmless, but a few signal that closer medical attention is needed.

- *Sturge-Weber Syndrome*
  When port wine stains involve the forehead and eyelid – and sometimes the cheek, nose and upper lip – there may be a risk of Sturge-Weber syndrome, which can be associated with seizures, learning difficulties, and glaucoma. Sturge-Weber syndrome is caused by abnormal blood vessels, often at the back of the brain in the occipital lobe. A brain scan, such as

an MRI, can clarify the extent of any affected areas. Treatment aims at modifying the symptoms. Laser treatment may be used to lighten or shrink the birthmark. Anticonvulsant medications may be prescribed to control seizures and brain surgery can produce excellent outcomes. Doctors recommend yearly monitoring for glaucoma and, again, surgery may be needed for this.

- *Klippel-Trenaunay-Weber syndrome*
  A port wine stain on an arm or leg may very occasionally indicate Klippel-Trenaunay-Weber syndrome, also called Parkes-Weber syndrome. As well as port wine stains – which are usually large – this is characterized by other blood vessel problems, such as varicose veins, and the overgrowth of soft tissue or bone, making one limb larger than the other. The effects range from mildly uncomfortable to severely disabling. While there is no cure, simple treatments may help, such as elastic compression stockings to reduce pain and swelling, laser therapy on the port wine stain itself and surgery for large marks or overgrown tissue. The syndrome has received some media attention due to the fact that US golfer Casey Martin has it.

Pigmented birthmarks

The colour of skin is created by melanin, a pigment produced by cells called melanocytes, of which there are typically between 1000 and 2000 per square millimetre of skin. Via a process called melanogenesis, melanocytes manufacture packets of melanin, called melanosomes, in the skin, eyes and hair.

Pigmented birthmarks are caused by an overgrowth of the cells that create pigment, so are composed of abnormal clusters of pigmented cells rather than the clusters of blood vessels that make up vascular birthmarks.

The commonest pigmented birthmarks are:

- cafe au lait spots

- Mongolian blue spots
- moles.

Some skin conditions that have an effect on skin pigmentation include:

- hyperpigmentation
- vitiligo
- melasma
- freckles.

Cafe au lait spots

These are light brown spots, often oval, that may be present at birth or appear a little later.

Many children have one or two of these and they are almost always harmless. If there are more than three or four, though, they should be checked by a doctor as they can occasionally mean that a child might have a rare disease, such as neurofibromatosis (a genetic disorder that causes abnormal cell growth of nerve tissues).

Mongolian blue spots

These are bluish, irregular flat patches, usually on the back and buttocks, though they can be on any part of the body.

They are very common in babies from ethnic groups who have darker skin colouring. They are harmless and become less obvious as the child grows.

Moles

Moles, or congenital nevi, are growths on the skin that usually are flesh-coloured, brown or black. They occur when cells in the skin grow in a cluster instead of being spread throughout the skin. These birthmarks are at a slight risk of developing into skin cancer, depending on their size, in which case they will be monitored and may be removed.

Treating pigmented birthmarks

Pigmented birthmarks usually do not need to be treated, with the exception of moles and, occasionally, cafe au lait spots.

Moles, especially if large, may be surgically removed. They should be monitored for life for any signs of growth or changes in shape or size, changes in colour or bleeding.

Cafe au lait spots can be removed with lasers, but tend to return.

Hyperpigmentation

Hyperpigmentation is a common, usually harmless, condition in which patches of skin become darker in colour. This is due to too much melanin being produced and forming deposits in the skin.

Age spots, usually on the hands and face, are a common form of hyperpigmentation. They occur due to sun damage and are referred to by doctors as solar lentigines.

Prescription creams can be used to lighten the skin, though they contain bleach or hydroquinone, which can irritate sensitive skin. Laser treatment may also help.

Vitiligo

Vitiligo, or leukoderma, is a chronic skin condition that causes loss of pigment or colour, resulting in irregular, pale patches of skin.

While the cause is complicated and not fully understood, there is some evidence to suggest that it is caused by a combination of autoimmune, genetic and environmental factors. Some genes can make people more susceptible to both vitiligo and some other autoimmune disorders, including a form of thyroid disease, type 2 diabetes, pernicious anaemia and others.

Vitiligo is estimated to affect at least 1 in every 100 people. It can begin at any age, though about 50 per cent of people with vitiligo develop it before the age of 25.

Skin affected by vitiligo is particularly vulnerable to sunlight because the melanocytes, which produce melanin and turn skin brown, are not active. It is therefore important to protect the skin with high-factor sunblock and protective clothing, not just to prevent the pain of sunburn but also because damage such as sunburn can stimulate the vitiligo to spread. Some brands of sunblock are classified by the NHS as borderline substances, which means that they can be obtained on prescription.

Treatments offered cannot cure vitiligo, but they can often slow its progress or, in some cases, bring about complete repigmentation. They include steroid creams, protopic cream (tacrolimus), and PUVA – a combination of medication (Psoralen) and treatment by ultraviolet A light. There is conflicting evidence about the effectiveness of laser treatments.

Melasma

Melasma usually takes the form of dark, irregular patches of skin, most frequently on the face.

Although it can affect anyone, melasma is particularly common in women, especially pregnant women, when it is also known as chloasma, or the mask of pregnancy. It is thought to be due to the hormones oestrogen and progesterone, which stimulate the production of melanocytes – the pigment-producing cells. It is also common in women taking oral contraceptives or HRT, those with light brown skin who live in sunny areas and those who have thyroid disease.

Melasma usually fades spontaneously over a period of months. If treatment is given its success is variable, but, whichever option is taken, it is important to protect the skin from sun. Bleaching creams containing hydroquinone can be tried, but should be used with caution as they can sometimes lead to increased and permanent darkening of the skin as well as being potentially irritating. A facial peel or cosmetic camouflage are other options.

Freckles

Though not strictly speaking classed as a birthmark or, indeed, a blemish, if they are numerous or very pronounced, freckles can sometimes cause distress.

There are several ways to treat freckles. Wearing a high-factor sunscreen can help block the sunlight that may darken freckles. A mild chemical peel can help to reduce the visibility of freckles. Bleaching creams may be effective in lightening some types of pigmentation or brown spots on the face, but can irritate sensitive skin. Laser treatment can sometimes be tried but the results are variable.

Vein disorders

Varicose veins and spider naevi

Vein disorders are common. Estimates vary, but they are believed to affect more than half of all women and around 45 per cent of men.

Varicose veins are enlarged veins that result from leaking valves and commonly appear as dilated, bulging and twisted rope-like veins under the skin. Veins have hundreds of one-way valves that help the blood flow in one direction, back to the heart. When these valves become damaged or diseased, blood migrates back towards the feet in response to gravity. The blood then pools in the veins and, where this happens, they appear dilated, bulging and twisted under the skin.

The veins in the legs and feet are the most commonly affected areas. This is because the legs have the most pressure from bodyweight, the force of gravity and the task of carrying the blood from the bottom of the body up to the heart.

Varicose veins arise as a result of defects in the valves within them that would normally prevent the backflow of blood that then pools. The tendency to have them is inherited. The hormonal changes associated with pregnancy can also be responsible as there is an increase in the volume of blood in the body, causing the veins to be swollen with extra fluid. This, combined with the pressure on the veins in the abdomen caused by the enlarged uterus, can cause swollen veins to turn into varicose ones. Other factors contributing to varicose veins include ageing, obesity, leg injury, a sedentary lifestyle, prolonged standing and exposure to the sun.

Spider naevi are smaller than varicose veins. These small, thin, spreading blood vessels (expanded capillaries), which are normally bright red, lie closer to the surface of the skin than do varicose veins, often on the face and chest, and become more noticeable in pregnancy. Spiders arise at this time because the capillaries expand under the influence of a rise in oestrogen levels, which is why they are prominent in pregnancy.

Spiders do not usually need medical treatment and are reasonably easy to cover with make-up. Varicose veins, however, as well as being unsightly, can become uncomfortable, causing swelling and pain. In some cases, varicose veins and spiders can cause more serious problems, such as venous insufficiency – a clogging of the blood in the veins that prevents it from returning to the heart. This, in turn can, though rarely, lead to problems such as a deep-vein thrombosis (blood clot) or infection, caused by an injury to the varicose vein, sores or skin ulcers.

Support stockings help your leg muscles push blood upwards and may relieve swelling and aching. They need to be worn all day and a proper fit is important, so do ask your GP or pharmacist for advice. Self-help measures include avoiding standing still for long periods of time, maintaining a healthy weight and taking regular exercise, such as walking. A high-fibre diet is also important, with plenty of fresh fruit and vegetables, to prevent constipation and straining at the toilet, which can worsen the state of the veins. Drinking plenty of water is also vital for the same reason.

Some complementary therapists suggest that eating a diet rich in vitamin C helps to strengthen blood vessels and that extra vitamin E might help to repair broken ones.

Surgery may be offered for very large veins. There are different operations, but the commonest is called ligation and stripping. This involves ligating (tying off) the vein so that the blood flow is cut off from it, then removing (stripping) part or all of it via a small cut in the skin.

Injection sclerotherapy is an alternative to surgery. This involves injecting veins with a chemical that seals the vein walls, creating scar tissue that closes off the affected vein. It may need to be done more than once.

Newer, minimally invasive treatments include laser surgery, microwave and radio frequency treatments. Endovenous ligation treatment (EVLT) is where a fine laser probe is passed inside a vein to heat and seal the vein.

Natural treatments include horse chestnut, witch hazel, used externally, Butcher's broom, grape seed and pine bark extracts. Consult your doctor before trying these. See also *Coping Successfully with Varicose Veins* by Christine Craggs-Hinton (Sheldon Press, 2007).

Rosacea

Rosacea is inflammation of parts of the face and may cause flushing, persistent facial redness (erythema), spots, eye problems and thickening of the skin. Rosacea is common, usually affecting those in middle or later life, and it is commoner in women and fair-haired people than the rest of the population.

Eye symptoms occur in more than half of cases, although they are often mild. They can include a feeling that there is something in the eye, burning or stinging, dryness, itching, sensitivity to light, blurred vision, eyelid cysts and styes and eyelid inflammation (blepharitis). Inflammation of the cornea (the front of the eye) is an uncommon but serious complication that can affect your vision. Do consult your doctor if you have any eye symptoms.

The exact cause of rosacea is not known, but it is thought that a number of factors may be involved, such as damage to the tiny blood vessels beneath the skin (usually from exposure to the sun), a mite called demodex follicularum and abnormal immune reactions in the skin.

While there is no cure, general self-help measures include avoiding strong sunlight and things that may make flushing worse, such as heat, alcohol, strenuous exercise, stressful situations, sunlight, spicy food or hot drinks. Fine laser treatment may also help (telangiectasia).

Lupus

Lupus is an autoimmune disorder that can affect almost any part of the body. It can cause different skin problems, the best-known of which is the characteristic red butterfly rash across the bridge of the nose and the cheeks. Other rashes can also occur on other parts of the body, ranging from widespread mild rashes to small distinct rashes on the elbows and knees. Specific problems include:

- discoid lupus, which usually affects the skin only and produces thickened, slightly red patches across the body
- subacute cutaneous lupus, which is a distinct rash that usually occurs in sun-exposed areas of the body, starting as scaly patches that increase in size with time
- panniculilis, which is inflammation of the fat below the skin, resulting in tender red lumps
- urticaria, which is an itchy, raised red rash, similar to nettle rash
- vasculitis, or inflamed blood vessels, which can cause painful red spots on the hands and feet and sometimes chilblain-type rashes; it can also occur in other areas of the body, affecting

internal organs such as the kidneys, and this needs to be treated very promptly.

Scars

Scars are tough bands of collagen, formed after injury to the skin. They are the skin's natural way of healing.

Scars may be formed for many different reasons, including as a result of infections, such as chickenpox, or surgery, injuries, burns or, in rare cases, by conditions such as scleroderma, where excessive amounts of collagen are deposited in the skin or other organs. Acne is another cause of scarring (see Chapter 2).

There are different types of scars. Some people – especially those with deeper skin tones – have a tendency to produce prominent, raised scars, called keloids. Stretchmarks (striae) are another type of scar that people may seek treatment for. These happen when the elastic layer of the skin under the surface is overstretched and the network of collagen and elastic fibres becomes weakened. There is no treatment that will reverse this once it has happened, but, with time, stretchmarks usually gradually improve. Laser treatment is sometimes tried, though it cannot eradicate the scarring and the final appearance will be identical to that of a mature stria – that is, a faded, silvery streak.

Scars generally do heal and fade naturally, but this process usually stops after around two years. That is why you may be advised to wait if you consult your doctor with a newer scar.

Massaging the skin with moisturizing creams may be helpful in speeding up the healing process and resulting in any scar being less visible. Some people recommend using a cream that has vitamin E in it (others feel that any moisturizing cream will work just as well) and ensuring that your diet is rich in vitamin E. Vitamin E is available in a variety of foods, particularly rich sources being most vegetable oils, margarine, wheatgerm, most nuts and leafy green vegetables. Sunblock is important if the scar is on exposed skin. Scars do not contain the normal pigments that protect skin and so they tend to burn easily.

There are several treatments that may be used to make scars flatter and smoother, depending on the type of scar in question, including steroid injections or applications and skin grafts. Silicon gel or gel sheets may help, but usually take at least two months before results become noticeable. They are available from some pharmacies. Drugs such as potassium aminobenzoate may help break down hardened scar tissue, while sometimes surgery is used to improve the appearance of scars in combination with or after other treatment methods. There is a growing trend for people to seek laser treatment for scars, which may improve the appearance of some scars, but is unlikely to remove them totally.

Ask your dermatologist, GP or pharmacist for further advice as the best type of treatment for you will depend on the type of scar you have. What may be suitable for an acne scar, for example, may not help with a keloid scar.

Tattoos

Despite their standing as modern fashion accessories, tattoos have been around for some time. The word 'tattoo' is derived from the Tahitian word 'tatau', meaning to mark, and the word 'tattaw' was first used in the 1769 account of Captain Cook's first voyage.

Tattoos, after the event, can be a cause of embarrassment or of downright emotional and psychological distress later on in life. They may sometimes come to be viewed in the same way as some people regard their birthmarks or scars – as a social nuisance or even a disfigurement.

There are several specific reasons for people wanting tattoos removed. One is that they are embarrassed about them –

especially if the tattoo contains a name, researchers have found. You may have outgrown the gang, true love or sentiments associated with the tattoo. Tattoos, among more conservative employers, are not deemed acceptable so they may make it difficult to get certain jobs or progress in your chosen career, especially if they can be interpreted as being rude, crude, racist, sexist, violent, intimidating or offensive in any other way.

Somewhat different are post-traumatic tattoos. These can be the result of a road traffic or other accident and are formed by ingrained dirt, such as from coal or tarmac, when wounds have been cleaned insufficiently. They tend to be bluish-black and may cause distress.

Medical tattoos are another special category. Examples are those used as markers in radiotherapy to ensure maximum accuracy for the treatment being given.

There are no official figures for how many people regret having their tattoos done, but the request for removal is generally agreed to be 'common'.

European missionaries in the Cook Islands tried to remove tattoos by scrubbing them off with sandstone – an uncomfortable form of treatment as the ink lies deep in the skin's dermis. Laser treatment is the treatment of choice for tattoos today as it carries a lower risk of scarring than earlier removal techniques, such as dermabrasion (where the surface and middle layers of skin are removed).

There are different types of laser treatment and the type used depends on the colours used in the tattoo. Colours that are easiest to remove are black, brown and blue, while red, green, yellow, orange and white are more difficult to remove. Generally, amateur tattoos are easier to remove than professional ones as the latter tend to include a wider variety of colours than amateur ones and no single laser can remove all the colours at the same time. Also, newer tattoos may contain more colouring than older ones, so it may take more treatment sessions to remove them than is necessary for older ones. Your age and skin type also influences the outcome of laser treatment.

2

Acne

I am devoting a whole chapter to acne – albeit a short one – because it is such a common problem and has such potentially severe psychological and emotional effects.

Acne affects more than 80 per cent of teenagers (those aged 13–18) at some point and it has been estimated that up to 30 per cent of teenagers have acne that is severe enough to require medical treatment. Acne can also persist into adulthood or, alternatively, strike for the first time in adults who escaped it in their teens. Indeed, the number of adults (those over the age of 25) with acne is increasing. The reasons for this increase are uncertain. Stress, environmental pollution, hormone-fed meat, increased exposure to the sun and hormonal fluctuations have all been cited as reasons, but some experts believe that people are simply more aware of acne or that the increase can be attributed to the fact that there are more people, as a result of the baby boom.

Acne is not classified as a disfigurement, but may be felt to be such by those who have it. How bad they think it is is often out of all proportion to its actual severity. As with other facial markings, acne can lead to low self-confidence, especially in the teenage years and young adulthood. Treatment does partly depend on the level of psychological distress experienced by the person, as well as how severe it may be, so, even if others tend to be dismissive, it is important to seek help from your doctor if it is bothering you.

The risk of scarring is another aspect that concerns people. About a quarter of those who suffer from acne between the ages of 12 and 24 will go on to have scars of varying severity. It is also known that adult acne is more likely to leave scars than is teenage acne. These do often fade with time – that is, after around 18 months to a couple of years – but it is obviously better to prevent them if you can by managing your acne as effectively as possible.

What is acne?

Acne – or acne vulgaris to give it its medical name – is a disorder of the sebaceous or oil glands. They become clogged up, causing pimples and inflammation on the face, chest, upper back or shoulders. What happens is that hormones called androgens stimulate the glands to increase oil production. The oil is broken down into free fatty acids by bacterial enzymes, which causes skin inflammation and abnormal plugging of the oil glands and hair follicles. Contrary to popular myth, this is not caused by poor diet or hygiene, although taking extra care in both these areas is likely to make acne easier to control.

Everyday care

Cleaning

While poor hygiene does not cause acne, it is important to keep the affected areas clean. Wash them twice a day (no more) with a mild soap or one that contains benzoyl peroxide. Do not scrub. For blackheads, a mild facial scrub will remove dead skin cells and dirt that can clog the pores. A clay mask is good and honey, raw if possible, has many antibacterial and antiseptic properties.

Here is some other useful advice.

- Once a week, steam your face for five minutes, having added a few drops of tea tree oil to boiling water.
- Keep long hair off the face and shoulders and wash it daily.

- Avoid shaving as much as possible. When you do, take care to avoid nicking the pimples and use a fresh razorblade to minimize the chance of spreading infection.
- Avoid make-up if possible or use only hypoallergenic or fragrance-free products.
- Do not pick the pimples – this may cause infection and scarring.
- Try over-the-counter treatments that contain substances such as benzoyl peroxide (gel or cream forms) or salicyclic acid. Start with the lowest strength and apply once a day about half an hour after washing. It may take several weeks to work. Never use more than 5 per cent strength without consulting a physician.
- Wash your pillowcase every other day as the fabric absorbs the dirt and oils from your skin and reapplies them to it as you sleep.

Diet and acne

Contrary to popular belief, it is generally agreed by doctors that acne is not caused by poor diet. However, eating a good, healthy diet, based on whole, unprocessed foods, can only benefit your general and skin health. Your skin is the largest organ of your body and, like other every other part of your body, needs proper nutrition in order to flourish.

Here are some general guidelines to eating healthily.

- Try to eat at least five portions of vegetables and at least one portion of fruit a day. Avoid anything white – refined flour, sugar – choosing wholegrain products instead.
- Avoid fats and fried foods, but do include foods containing omega 3, such as flax seeds, and oily fish, such as sardines, mackerel and salmon. Other sources include soya, walnuts and dark green leafy vegetables.

- Some people find that chocolate, caffeine, fizzy drinks, shellfish, wheat and/or milk products make their acne worse.
- Drink plenty of water every day – in the form of tap or mineral water, fruit juice and herbal teas. Do not forget, soup can be a source of water and vegetables at the same time. It is a good idea to drink water with soup, however, especially if the soup is salty.

Regular bowel movements are important. The above measures should ensure regularity, but if not, in addition try dried fruit, such as prunes, apricots and figs, or a teaspoon of linseed or flax seeds twice a day.

Vitamins and minerals

Certain vitamins and minerals have been suggested as being helpful in relation to acne and general skin health. It is usually best to try and increase your intake of these from food sources rather than take supplements, especially with vitamin A as high doses of this vitamin carry a risk of decreased bone density, birth defects, headaches and muscle and joint pain.

Vitamin A

Increasing your intake may help to reduce sebum production, but it is best not to take supplements as too high a dose can be toxic. Instead, obtain vitamin A in the form of carotene from food sources such as carrots, pumpkin, cantaloupe and other yellow-orange fruits and vegetables. Liver, eggs and whole milk are also good sources of vitamin A, as are fortified cereals and bread.

Decreasing your intake of unhealthy fats, such as margarine, hydrogenated oils and processed foods, can also improve the body's absorption of vitamin A.

Zinc

Zinc may help reduce inflammation and promote skin healing. Food sources include red meat, seafood such as oysters, liver, whole grains, pulses and legumes, eggs, almonds and Brazil nuts, pumpkin seeds, milk and dairy products.

Vitamin B6

This vitamin may help premenstrual or mid-cycle acne as it plays a role in controlling the sex hormones as well as being important for healthy skin and hair.

Vitamin B6 can be found in whole grains, dairy foods, red meat, oily fish, eggs, green leafy vegetables and beans and peas.

Chromium

Chromium is thought to work with insulin to regulate blood sugar. Some studies suggest that unstable blood sugar levels may be linked with severe acne, which can be relieved by ensuring that you have extra chromium in the form of yeast.

This is an area that needs more research and, as with other supplements, it is best to source chromium from food such as brewer's yeast, liver and other meat, whole grains, wheatgerm, lentils and spices, rather than take it in tablet form.

Complementary remedies

The following are complementary remedies that some people have found helpful, though they should not preclude other, more conventional means of treatment. Consult your doctor or a qualified practitioner for individual guidance or if you are in any doubt as to whether or not you should try these.

Herbal medicine

Some remedies that have been recommended for acne include blackcurrant seed oil or evening primrose oil, echinacea, calendula and goldenseal.

Sarsaparilla, yellow dock, burdock and cleavers, mixed together in equal measures, are believed to be potent blood and lymph cleansers.

The ancient Egyptians used poultices of wet strawberry leaves to improve the complexion.

Essential oils

Essential oils may be applied topically to skin for mild to moderate acne. Be sure to follow the directions on the bottle, and to dilute the oil if directed to do so; as a general rule, the more sensitive your skin is, the more diluted the oil should be. Mix a few drops with a carrier oil such as grapeseed, or with witch hazel, and dab gently on to skin; do not massage if your skin is inflamed, and cease use if irritation develops. Tea tree oil, a natural antiseptic and anti-bacterial, is most commonly recommended for acne, and other oils used include lavender oil, bergamot and geranium.

What makes acne worse?

- The menstrual cycle – acne often worsens just before a period or in mid cycle.
- Prescription medication, such as certain birth control pills, steroids and lithium.
- Being overweight – increased insulin production can signal to the body to release extra male hormones, androgens, which are involved in pimple formation.
- Stress.
- Cosmetics, sunscreen, moisturizers, grease and oil in products – all clog the pores.
- Although no link has been found between chocolate intake and acne, some people find that certain foods do make their acne worse, such as chocolate, sugar, fats, fried, salty and processed foods, caffeine, fizzy drinks, dairy products and seafood and other iodine-rich foods.
- Not enough water, healthy oils, fruit and vegetables or fibre – constipation can also worsen acne.

- Tumours in the adrenal glands and polycystic ovary syndrome.

Treatments

Treatments divide into those you can buy over the counter and those that can be prescribed by your doctor.

Effectiveness of over-the-counter products

Scientists at the universities of Nottingham and Leeds have found that some of the cheapest acne treatments available on the high street are more effective than antibiotics (M. Ozolins, et al., 'Comparison of five antimicrobial regimens for treatment of mild to moderate inflammatory facial acne vulgaris in the community: randomised controlled trial', *The Lancet*, 18/25 December 2004, 364, pp. 2188–95). Professor Tony Avery and colleagues conducted a study into facial acne, which revealed that cheap, topical acne treatments are just as effective as antibiotics and should be used as a first choice to save money and reduce bacterial resistance – an important consideration given concerns about this happening as a result of the overuse of antibiotics.

Over-the-counter products

Over-the-counter products are best used for mild acne. They may take a few weeks to work, so, if you do not see any improvement after a couple of months or if your acne worsens, do consult your doctor.

Products available from your local pharmacy often contain benzoyl peroxide, which is an antibacterial agent. It attacks the bacteria that cause inflammation in acne. It can also clear blocked pores and has a drying effect on skin. A common side-effect is mild skin irritation.

Prescription treatments

Your GP may also prescribe benzoyl peroxide. If this does not work or you have more severe acne, other treatments include creams to rub into the skin, which tend to be for less severe acne, or tablets to take orally.

Creams include azelaic acid and retinoids, which both work to unblock clogged pores. Retinoids can cause skin irritation and should not be used if you are pregnant or planning to become pregnant – do tell your doctor if this is the case.

Oral medications include antibiotics to kill off the bacteria and reduce inflammation, which may be used together with a cream that helps unblock pores. It may take a few weeks before any improvement becomes noticeable.

Some oral contraceptive tablets help clear up acne in women. The main point is that you do not have to just put up with acne, believing that nothing can be done. Have a chat with your doctor to find out the best options for you and, whatever treatment is decided on, do bear in mind that you need to persevere with it – a common reason for persistent acne is giving up a treatment too soon. Check with your doctor or pharmacist how long it takes for a treatment to work and give it a chance before switching to another one.

Treatments for scarring

Some people are more prone to scarring than others because of genetic predisposition or skin colour. There are two types of acne scars:

- pigmented scars, which leave behind a purplish-brown mark once the blemish has gone away
- ice pick scars, which leave a small depression in the skin.

Time is one of the best treatments for acne scars, which, like other scars, do improve over a period of several months. Otherwise, laser treatments, dermabrasion and chemical peels have all been suggested for scarring, though none will remove all traces. Laser treatment tends to be more successful with milder scarring, less so with the deeper scars. Anyone thinking about this form of treatment should discuss the risks with their doctor, such as infection, including herpes, recurrent acne, changes in skin pigmentation and inflammation.

3

Like your look

I walked on to the platform for the Tube and there she was, staring straight at me, hugely larger than life: a poster of a stunningly attractive model with a prominent, bright birthmark around her right eye. It was brighter and more noticeable than any mark I had ever seen. In fact, it seemed to glisten … it did glisten. It was not a birthmark at all, I quickly realized – it was a clever piece of asymmetrical make-up, designed to stun the viewer with an unusual and arresting vision of attractiveness. In essence, though, this artificial facial feature was no different in its form from many natural features, such as birthmarks. Because it was intended to be surprising and attractive, I took it as such. If it had not been make-up, would I have been able to see it in the same attractive light?

In the Introduction, we explored the idea that our faces are intimately linked to how we see ourselves and imagine others see us. However, this does not simply happen 'to' us, it is something that we are part of. We make choices and allow ourselves to be influenced by ideas of beauty and normality, visions of the ideal and ideas about what is 'ugly'.

Beverley Fulker, who set up Love Your Mark – a collection of inspirational stories about people living happily and successfully with their birthmarks and scars – is someone who has considered this issue in relation to her facial birthmark and has come to a conclusion that some might find surprising. Here is Beverley's story in her own words as told on her website, Love Your Mark (www.loveyourmark.com):

Be different and be happy!

I am a life coach and mentor and I specialize in helping people with marks, scars and facial differences. I hope I can inspire others to be happy with themselves.

As a child, I would have been ecstatic if I had been able to meet others with birthmarks. It would have given me great encouragement and confidence. I went through a phase of asking for plastic surgery but now I am glad my parents talked me out of it. I have a facial port wine stain and have had a happy life – a little teasing when I was young but nothing terrible – without any counselling.

In 2003, I saw a documentary which changed my life. I was sad to learn that there are so many people with marks and scars who are unhappy. I had always been interested in helping people and, in particular, in confidence building, so I decided to become a mentor and try to help others gain confidence and learn to live happily with their differences.

I was lucky to have loving parents and I never gave my mark much thought until I was teased, aged eight. Then I wanted to hide my mark and I used camouflage make-up for years. It seems strange to look back, now that I don't wear make-up, but when I went to the office I always covered it with make-up, as I thought that would be more 'professional'!

Now I realize that most people are perfectly accepting and there is no need to feel paranoid. Many people have 'irrational beliefs' about their scars and marks. However, we are humans and scars and marks are only natural and we should not have to hide them. I threw my make-up away in April 2004 and feel really good about that! Freedom!

Beverley has made a conscious decision that her mark is part of her face, that it is natural and not something to hide or attempt to remove. She is clearly able to empathize with others who may not be so positive about their faces, for whatever reason, and this has led her to develop a coaching and mentoring service that aims to help others to overcome negative feelings about their faces.

Two things stand out strongly for me in Beverley's brief biography. The first is the vital role that her parents played in encouraging a positive and healthy attitude to her face. It is clear that this was part of an affirming upbringing, summed up in the simple phrase, 'I was lucky to have loving parents'. Lucky indeed and it is clear that this has given Beverley a solid bedrock for her positive outlook on life. She is also fortunate that she only experienced 'a little teasing when I was young but nothing terrible', as others have had much worse experiences that make it harder for them to be positive about their faces. However, the word 'fortunate' might not be the most appropriate word as, to some extent, we make our own luck and I have no doubt that the young Beverley was able to cope with teasing and attract less of it precisely because of her loving background and positive self-image. There is more about this and related issues in Chapters 6 and 7.

The second phrase that stands out for me is, 'Many people have "irrational beliefs" about their scars and marks.' This seems to me to be crucial. If you have a facial feature you feel uncomfortable about, is it really rational to say that it stops you from doing something? Does it have the ability to tell you, 'Sorry, you can't go there' or 'I'm afraid you can't do that'? Clearly it does not, yet many of us allow ourselves to think in this way. We may not articulate the thought, but, if you dig beneath the surface of your thinking, you might find thoughts along the lines of, 'If only it wasn't for my mark/scar/facial feature, I'd be able to …'.

Here are some simple thought experiments and exercises for anyone who has a facial feature they feel uncomfortable about. My aim is to help you uncover the sorts of irrational beliefs that Beverley identifies, then work on them in a more rational way.

If you are new to these kinds of imaginative exercises and find them a little strange, simply read through them and try to get a picture of what they are aiming at. Then, pluck up the courage to give one a go. They are totally private so no one else need know. If you find that a particular exercise is not for you, devise your own version by thinking through the questions that the exercises are asking and then find your own ways to answer them in your head or by writing or drawing your responses. There are similar exercises for parents and children in Chapter 7.

Exercise 1: Name your mark!

Give your mark or other facial feature a name. Try to think of something appropriate, something that reflects how you tend to think and feel about it. So, if, like Beverley, you have learned to love your mark, you might choose a name that reflects qualities of love and friendship, such as Amy, Grace, Hope or Aamir ('full of life'). Alternatively, you might choose a name with a less positive feel, such as ugly Betty or angry Alan. You can choose a name that has particular connotations for you, reminding you of a particular person, positive or negative. You might, of course, simply go for the neutral 'Mark', although to me this does not seem entirely neutral as, in the context, you are naming something after its form, rather like calling your cat 'cat', so it could suggest a lack of warmth in your feelings towards your mark.

You can extend this exercise by not limiting yourself to actual names, but giving your thoughts free rein to come up with descriptive words or phrases that could refer back to childhood nicknames or simply seem to you to encapsulate how you feel about your mark. In my case, as mentioned earlier, it would be Blotch or Belisha Beacon.

Take your time with this exercise. I find that I get the best out of this sort of thing if I find time for some relaxed thinking – what some might call meditation. I have to take occasional train journeys and they are ideal for this. I find that if I allow myself a few minutes to relax, close my eyes, do some deep breathing and then let my thoughts gently focus on the issue, I produce a much more considered set of ideas than I would if I sat down with pen and paper.

You might have your own preferences – liking to do your thinking on paper or while out walking or in the bath, for example. Choose whatever works for you. There are lots of tips for relaxation, meditation and visualization in my book *The Confidence Book* (Sheldon Press, 2007) and its accompanying website The Confidence Site (www.theconfidencesite. co.uk).

Exercise 2: What's in a name?

You have now given your mark a name. This exercise helps you to think a little more deeply about how you feel about it.

Imagine that, now it has a name, your mark also has a personality. How would you describe it?

The first example below takes the form of a spoof biography of a birthmark. This is one approach and it might suit you, but you can try this exercise in any way that fits your style. You might like to write a simple list or prefer to write a poem or do an annotated drawing. Examples of each follow.

Biography
Violet has changed over the years. When I was young, she was a quiet girl, following me around and so timid that I hardly knew she was there.

Later, in adolescence, she began to assert herself and at times seemed to gain an 'n' as she moved beyond assertiveness into being quite demanding. She'd shout 'Look at me' all the time and I began to feel that our positions were reversed. She was the one everyone was noticing and I felt like her side-kick. It was not a pleasant experience.

Violet has calmed down now, but she still seems to take the lead sometimes, particularly when I find myself with a group of strangers. I'm sure they're all giving Violet more attention than they're giving me.

List
Name: Bigfoot
Age: 37 – shares my exact birthday!
Education: School of hard knocks.
Health: Has diminished over the years (laser treatment).
Qualities: Now often hides (behind camouflage). Can be angry, vivid, attention-seeking.

Poem
I am: all can see
Bright beacon – pay heed to me
One leaf – not whole tree.

This is a dialogue between an aggressive mark and someone with a greater sense of perspective. Creativity often works best if you give yourself some sort of structure, so you could try a five-, seven-, five-syllable approach as above or a dialogue poem or an acrostic (the first letter of each line forming the name you have given your mark, for example). Why not give it a go and see if it helps you to think through your beliefs and attitudes about your mark?

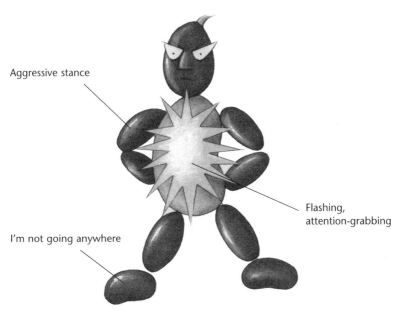

Aggressive stance

Flashing, attention-grabbing

I'm not going anywhere

Purple Meanie Beanie Man!

You might be someone who finds this way of thinking enjoyable and helpful or you might prefer a more straightforward approach. What is important is that, however you get there, you come out of this exercise with an understanding of how you think about the facial feature that you are working on. What are the underlying beliefs that you have about it? Are they mostly positive, negative, a mixture of the two or mostly indifferent?

To end this exercise, write a brief summary of your thoughts and feelings about your mark. This part of the exercise will particularly suit those who prefer a straightforward approach, but for those who value the imaginative exercises, it can ground your thinking and make your thoughts more acute. Here is an example of the kind of thing you might write at this point: 'I think of my birthmark less now than I used to, but I am still conscious of it in a negative way, thinking of it as something that holds me back by making me feel different, unusual and odd.'

Finally in this section, a challenge: can you find positive ways to think about your facial feature?

Acknowledge any negative thoughts that you may have explored above, but try now to see these in context. So, for example, you might create a list like the following.

- Bert (name given to mark in Exercise 1) doesn't do any actual harm. He isn't disabling in any way.
- Bert is part of me and I need to learn to be positive about every aspect of myself.
- Bert makes me distinctive.
- If I find Bert's distinctness difficult, then this spurs me on to be more outgoing, to show people that I have a lot of positive things going for me.
- My family (or lover/children/friends …) love me, so Bert can't be a barrier to what really matters.
- Bert doesn't stop me doing anything that I want to do.

Exercise 3: Some may say …

Have you ever heard any direct comments about your mark or facial feature, apart from in a medical or cosmetic context?

In my research, I have discovered that some people with birthmarks have been unfortunate enough to overhear derogatory comments ranging from (to a child), 'Don't stare at that lady's odd face' to 'Urghh, did you see that?' Some have even been directly confronted with suggestions that they should not be out looking like that.

It may be painful, but, if you can, write down any actual overheard or direct comments about your facial feature. Give some context – was it direct or overheard, what were the ages of the people, what was the tone? As an example, here are three of my memories.

- At school, aged 13, my 'friend' – this is just one of many examples of things said when I walked into a room: 'Aagghh, it's so bright, turn that beacon down …'.
- Overheard in the street about five years ago, a couple of teenage boys were giggling: 'God, did you see that man's face? God!'
- In Lewisham, again about five years ago, I was approached by a very friendly guy: 'You want some weed for that, man? Good-quality weed soon get rid of that for you …'.

How do you react to your own memories? Are they painful for you or do you have a sense of perspective that helps you to see them in a wider context? Choose a couple of comments, if you have them, and write down your reactions beside them, like this.

- Overheard in the street about five years ago, a couple of teenage boys were giggling: 'God, did you see that man's face? God!'
  They are adolescents and find anything out of the ordinary threatening.

If they had not found my birthmark to laugh at they would have found something else and, if not me, someone else. It wasn't personal, it was just them.

- In Lewisham, again about five years ago, I was approached by a very friendly guy: 'You want some weed for that, man? Good-quality weed soon get rid of that for you …'.

  I laughed about this at the time and still do. It was a surreal but pleasant conversation and, when he realized that I was not buying, we parted with a smile. It was the first, and last, time that I heard of cannabis being a cure for birthmarks!

So you can see that, in my case, I have been able to put these events into proper perspective and be calm and not upset by them. My attitude is that there will always be cruel and unpleasant people, those who will find fault with anyone who is different from them. If it were not a facial feature, it would be something else. The human race loves the safety of sameness and some people will hit out at anything that threatens their limited ideas about what is 'normal'. I also accept that, in the case of young people, many will 'grow out of it'.

This is not to say that words and aggressive reactions, particularly from groups, cannot hurt us. Some people say that they can diminish our positive sense of self and sap our confidence. Actually, they can't. Words can do nothing unless we let them. It is our reactions that are the 'hurt'. We may feel that we have good reason to be upset, we may believe that it is appropriate to feel this way, but this does not detract from the simple fact that the hurt lies in our reaction, not in the words themselves.

Let me give a quick illustration of this. Suppose I said to you, 'You have the brain of a gnat and even the gnat was glad to get rid of it.' These are, of course, just words. They can't make you feel anything – how could they? I do not know you, so I have no basis for my insult whatsoever. If you did react negatively to those words, it was your doing and that would also be the case if someone you knew made that comment and even if you respected him or her. The words themselves have no power – your reaction does.

Having established that this is so, it does not mean that it is an easy or a non-problem – far from it. Our reactions can be difficult to tame. I believe that the way to deal with these kinds of thoughts is put them into perspective, to try and understand why the comment was made and why you reacted as you did. It is an issue of confidence, one of being prepared to do some work on your thoughts and feelings. It is a matter of allowing yourself to stand up to negativity and replace it with a more confident understanding.

If you have had negative reactions to anything you have written in the course of this exercise, go back over it and write – in a different colour (or on a new piece of paper if it is getting too messy) – a more considered and positive approach based on a more balanced perspective and the following key messages:

- words do not hurt
- the hurt lies in my reaction
- people often say things out of ignorance
- people have an instinct to herd together in safe groups with those similar to them
- I am not defined by the reactions of others
- I am not perfect, either within or without, but I can be happy with who I am
- I am a 'work in progress' and my positive sense of self is developing all the time.

If you find any of this difficult, remember that coaching is available, so you might like to seek out either a professional coach or a trusted friend to help you think things through in a positive light.

Exercise 4: Some may think ...

Having looked at what people say, we shall move on now to the trickier area of what they think.

The truth is, we can never know what people really think, even if we believe what they are telling us. In my improvization classes, we do a simple exercise in which people, after they have said something, say what they are actually thinking. For example:

Darling, I've been so looking forward to seeing you. (Oh no, I've got to tell her.)
You look great. (Couldn't you have made an effort?)
I've got something to tell you. (Be brave, here goes, tell her: it's over.)
I saw Julie the other day. (Why did I say that? What a wimp – just tell her!)

The essential point is that we often think we know what people are thinking, but, in fact, it is a story that we are telling ourselves. No end of confusion arises from our reactions to things that no one has said and probably no one is thinking either. So, if you have negative thoughts about a facial feature, are these based on what you imagine people's reactions to be rather than what they actually think? Try the following exercise.

- Track your thoughts about your facial feature during the day.
- Note down any reactions that you seem to pick up from other people – things that you interpret from their tone of voice, looks and facial expressions.
- Then, in each case, see if you can think of an alternative explanation.

Here are a couple of examples.

- I entered the room and a stranger stared.
  - *Interpretation* She was staring at my birthmark.
  - *Alternative interpretations* She was trying to remember if she knew me, I reminded her of someone, she was having a 'vacant moment', she fancied me.
- As I left, two women were engaged in a whispered conversation. One glanced at me and quickly looked away.
  - *Interpretation* They were commenting on my mark and wondering how I could go out looking like that.
  - *Alternative interpretations* They were talking about someone and did not want me to hear, they need to ask me something and are plucking up courage, they are sharing a risqué joke.

Do you always accept the least positive interpretation of what you think others are thinking? Do you tend to let your facial feature dominate your thoughts and think that it is what others most notice about you, too? Be really honest, do you always interpret glances and expressions as being about you?

You can see how easy it is to get the wrong impression when you begin to imagine the thoughts of others. The answer to this is the same as it was for Exercise 3 – we have to put things into proper perspective.

The following is a list of what I think happened when I met new people in the days before I started using camouflage make-up.

- *Stage 1* Probably the first thing they noticed was my birthmark. It made me stand out and was, of course, noticeable.
- *Stage 2* As we talked, they formed a more rounded opinion of me. Whether they liked me or not is immaterial here. The point is that they began to see the whole person and my mark was assimilated into their 'whole picture', no longer worth noting.
- *Stage 3* If we met again, they might notice my mark afresh because they had forgotten about it, which indicates how unimportant it was to the bigger picture. On this second meeting, they would assimilate it even more quickly into their overall view of me than they did the first time.

This tells me pretty clearly that any problems I had with how I looked and my decision to use camouflage were based not on others and their views, but on me and how I viewed myself. You can read more about this in Chapter 4, Camouflage.

Thus, if you can gain a true picture of what you think about your facial feature, what others say and what you think they think, then you are in a much stronger position to make informed decisions about your options for treatment or, like Beverley, see that you can love your mark and be proud of your distinctiveness.

I want to end this chapter with the words of Mike, one of Beverley's friends, quoted on her website. I think he sums up many of the issues we have been looking at.

> I'm a pretty happy guy and I rarely think about my birthmark – at least not in any sort of detrimental fashion. I'm just me, it's there, it always has been and, in some form or another, always will be. This is how I am supposed to be, this is life, and it suits me just fine.
>
> Generally, though ... I don't see anything strange or different or odd or out of place when I look in the mirror. I just see me. My friends and family feel the same. They've told me this many times, and often I found it hard to believe, but as life goes on I meet more and more people who say something like: 'Oh, after meeting you a couple times I didn't even think about it any more.' So I guess it must be true. Regardless, it is nice to know that people view others by what's on the inside more often than they do otherwise.
>
> My birthmark isn't very big and coincidentally looks like a black eye, or so strangers often remark. I've had about seven or eight laser treatments now and it has faded considerably. My doc says 50 per cent, but that was before the last two zaps. I'm pleased with that. It's lighter, smoother-looking, and generally softer in appearance. Rarely do I ever encounter anyone who is clearly distressed over it. Local cashiers who see me all the time have figured it out by now. Once in a while I'll notice some stares or run into a few less educated individuals who find it hard to look me in the eye when we have to communicate, but this is very rare indeed. Mostly ... I feel like any other normal, ordinary, average guy.

I go for laser treatments mostly just because I *can*. It is afford-able and effective these days. I am always on the lookout for ways in which to improve myself in all areas: mental, physical, spiritual, emotional, intellectual, etc. I use Crest Whitestrips on my teeth once a year also simply because I *can*. It's something just for *me*, not for anyone else. I feel good about *caring* for myself, you know? I think of the laser treatments in the same way. It's for me, because I can. In a way, oddly, I am sort of glad that an argon laser treatment, when I was about 13 years old, left some mod-erate, residual scarring. If today's lasers continue to improve and one day in the future I *do* find that I can get most of the colour out ... I think I'd be sad to see it all go! A little bit of off-colour tissue under my eye ... well, it just feels like that is *supposed* to be there.

Whatever kind of man I am right now and whatever I may grow in spirit to be in the future, my birthmark has helped make me who I am. My life might have been different without it – I may have not been able to see things from the perspective of someone who is unique in a physical way. So I'm glad I have that silly mark. I think it's OK to improve it, just as long as I don't ever forget it.

4

Camouflage

To camouflage something is to create an illusion of invisibility. For example, a soldier's camouflage clothing does not actually hide him or her, but tricks the watching eye by making the soldier blend into the background with similar shades and patterns to those of the terrain, whether forest or desert. An even more subtle form of camouflage is the use of lighting, a technique that goes back to World War II when some allied aircraft used lights tuned to the luminescence of the sky to make them disappear. Effectively, to an observer on the ground or at sea, the aircraft would not stand out against the background of the sky because they shone with light of the same intensity.

The key point to notice about any type of camouflage is that it does not have to blend in perfectly. Soldiers' clothing does not match the background exactly, nor has someone copied the exact flora of each area and applied these images to the clothing. The lights on the World War II aircraft did not create anything like a high-definition picture of the sky they were seen against. If something does not stand out to you, if you do not notice it, then it is invisible. Thus, all that is needed for camouflage to be successful is that it tricks the eye.

This is the principle behind the use of camouflage make-up to cover birthmarks and other facial blemishes. In the UK, the camouflage service is run by the British Red Cross (<www .redcross.org.uk>) and it has people who teach those with certain skin conditions and scars how to use long-lasting, waterproof cover creams that are available on the NHS. It stresses that the creams are not make-up in the conventional sense as they are applied to conceal only the affected area (but see the section headed 'All over?' later in this chapter). They are appropriate for men, women and children and can be used on other parts of the body as well as the face.

The Red Cross recommends the creams for disguising such conditions as:

- vitiligo
- rosacea and lupus
- spider naevi
- birthmarks
- hyperpigmentation
- scars
- burns
- leg veins
- tattoos.

They carry demonstration stocks of products by all the major manufacturers in hundreds of shades. You can get information on the clinic nearest to you from the Red Cross website given above, but you will need to be referred by your doctor.

My own story

Camouflage was the route I went down only relatively late in life. You might wonder why I waited so long to think about getting something done about my birthmark. My decision coincided with a number of changes in my life, including leaving the BBC in 2001, where I'd been a producer since 1989, in order to freelance. This has led to an interesting mix of work and one aspect is that I've discovered I really enjoy, and seem to be reasonably good at, training and development. I run a wide range of courses and events that all require me to introduce myself to groups of strangers. Whether it takes seven seconds or not, first impressions do count to some extent and I realized that I didn't want people to be sizing me up by my birthmark rather than by what I was saying.

Maybe I wanted a way to mark my new beginning. Anyway, I plucked up some courage and made an appointment with my doctor. Why did this take courage? First, I'm part of that large subsection of the male population who feels that they can only go to the doctor if there is a very good reason. Second, I am quite reserved about discussing personal things. My wife was a great help, practical as ever, and the appointment was made.

My doctor completely understood and went through the options. She was very clear about the visibility of my birthmark, describing it as 'vivid' and 'angry'. This didn't upset me at all – in fact, seeing my birthmark through her eyes gave me a strong sense that I was doing the right thing.

It wasn't long before I had an appointment at a hospital in London to see a consultant. As it is a teaching hospital, I was asked if someone could sit in on the consultation, then someone else joined in, so there was the consultant himself and three other medical staff or trainees, all having a good look at my vivid, angry birthmark.

I elected not to have laser treatment when it was offered. It didn't take me long to reach this decision. There were two main reasons for it. First, it was explained to me that, in my case, the effectiveness was likely to be towards the lower end of the scale. This was because I had 'presented' late (a polite way of saying that I was getting on a bit) and thus my mark had thickened to a deep purple. There would definitely be a noticeable improvement, but I was likely to need to use camouflage cream over what remained. Second, there would have to be several treatment sessions and bruising would follow each one. As after all this I would probably still have to use make-up afterwards anyway, I decided not to go ahead with laser treatment.

This was a very personal decision and I would not want to put anyone off from exploring the laser option. It is a major and highly effective form of permanent treatment and, particularly when used on the young, can mean that many people forget their mark entirely or have its impact severely diminished.

So, I went to the Red Cross for my first lesson in applying camouflage make-up with some trepidation. I am a man and make-up, even if you call it camouflage cream, is not usually part of my world. I do some acting, but that's different. The idea of putting on make-up and walking down the street made me feel very uncomfortable.

I met two friendly women nurses and we had a brief chat, but all the while I was aware that my eyes kept straying towards the table full of brushes, wipes and camouflage samples – samples that, despite what the Red Cross says on its website, looked suspiciously like make-up to me.

I don't see anything intrinsically wrong with men wearing make-up, it's just not something that I would normally do or feel comfortable with. I had a barrier to get over, an association of camouflage with make-up and of make-up with the feminine. At the same time, there was a curiosity and a sense of fun, of playing and trying something new.

The Red Cross nurses started matching shades to my skin colour and we soon decided that a mix of two shades was needed. I now think this was a blessing as skin colour varies throughout the year and with two shades you can adjust the mix to match it as it changes. We tried one combination, but on my skin it looked grey. Although the colour looked pretty good on the palette, it looked wrong on my skin. The colours can look different depending on where you see them, the background they're against and the lighting conditions, so you need to experiment.

We tried again and, although I had my reservations, the Red Cross nurses assured me that it was a very good match and people would not notice it. I wanted my birthmark to disappear under perfect make-up, but this could never happen for me as I know where to look and so will always spot the patch of more even colour without the freckles and minor imperfections of real skin. Someone else, who wasn't looking for it, wouldn't see it, though. This was demonstrated almost at once as a student nurse arrived. She couldn't see where it was until it was pointed out to her.

I had a bit a of a shock a few moments later as I was removing the make-up in order to have a go myself (removing make-up was another new skill for me). As I wiped it off, I saw the student nurse wince – that vivid, angry mark, suddenly revealed, had come as a surprise to her.

I practised putting the creams on myself twice. The whole session lasted about an hour, including completing the paperwork to get my new prescriptions. I didn't want to go home on the train wearing make-up, even if it was called cream and pretending to be medical rather than cosmetic. I said that I would take it off and try it later, but I was persuaded to leave it on to try it out and so I did. How strange that I should feel so self-conscious about being seen *without* my birthmark. Of course, no one stared at me and, when I got home, my wife was amazed at the result. From then on, I was hooked.

Bridget just says no!

Bridget Crawshaw is a contact made via the Birthmark Support Group (www.birthmarksupportgroup.org.uk); here's what she had to say about hospital visits with several staff present, as reported in *The Confidence Book* (Sheldon Press, 2007):

There was one particular incident at a hospital check-up when I was little that is imprinted in my mind. I remember being called in to see the plastic surgeon and when I walked in there he was behind his desk and behind him a row of trainees; it was awful. I endured the usual prodding and poking and was stared at by all these people. I can't remember whether we were even given the option of whether we wanted them there or not or even how many there were but to a small child and in my mind now there were too many!

This may seem insignificant to some but each time I was in hospital, and the team of doctors would come round to look, I wanted to curl up and die.

I am certain that that day has had a big impact on my behaviour. I think up to a point when you are little that you are oblivious and your parents are going through hell and then you become aware that things are not exactly how they should be!

Now if I've been in a doctor's surgery or wherever and I get asked if I mind students being present I say yes and ask them to leave (but then feel bad!)

I do not think Bridget should feel bad about this – it is perfectly reasonable to want your consultation to be as private as possible and members of the medical profession recognize this, which is why they ask the question.

Camouflage tips

Órla Checksfield coordinates the adult section of the Birthmark Support Group. Her expertise and positive character have been a great help to me as I have put this book together, both in terms of her own comments and putting me in touch with a number of other people whose stories and tips appear in this book. Órla has contributed substantially to the following tips.

Find your make-up

There are several manufacturers of camouflage creams, each with their own formulations, ranges of shades and fixing powder (see below). It is usually easier to get all your supplies from one manufacturer, but this is not the only consideration. You may end up with, say, a cream and powder from one manufacturer and another cream of a different make because they give you the best colour blend.

Here are some other points to consider.

- Does the cream cause you any irritation or other skin problems?
- Is it readily available?
- What does it cost (if you are paying for it yourself rather than getting it on prescription)?
- Is it available in sufficiently large tubs to give you a good supply?

I can attest to the importance of the second and fourth considerations. A couple of years ago, my local pharmacy was no longer able to supply the range that I had been using. There was a complicated story regarding some corporate decisions being made about supplying the NHS that meant, in the future, the brand would only be available from a few pharmacies. When I called in at the nearest of these, which meant a trip to London (as I often work there, it was not a problem, but it could have been for other people), the pharmacy had no supplies. When it finally did get some a few weeks later, all it had were tiny pots containing less than a quarter of the amount I usually had. My doctor organized another visit to the Red Cross camouflage clinic for me and I switched to another range of products, which, luckily, suit me very well. The moral of this story is that there are practical considerations as well as medical and cosmetic ones.

In the UK, through your GP, make an appointment at a Red Cross camouflage clinic if you can. Another route, which may be better for you if you live in another country, is to explore the websites of organizations concerned with your condition. There you can see what other people who use camouflage creams do, which brands they use and so on, then take a look at the various manufacturers' websites. Many offer samples so you can try out a selection of shades at home to find what suits you best. Also, some beauticians stock and demonstrate camouflage make-up.

Once you have found your colour match, you can go back to your GP and organize getting the creams on prescription.

Find your application method

The Red Cross nurses teach people how to use a palette and brushes to apply the creams. This gives the smoothest results and avoids mixing oils from the hands into the creams.

Some people find the following method works better for them. Mix the colours in the palm of your right hand, using the fingertips of your left hand, and then apply the blended creams.

You will need to experiment to find which method works best for you.

Any cream and all methods require you to start with clean skin. It is recommended that you use make-up remover to clean the skin first, then an astringent designed to remove any remaining traces of make-up, dirt and oil without drying the skin. I gave up using the astringent after a while, though, as it just seemed too much hassle in the morning and I seem to be getting along just fine without it. Some people use make-up removing wipes to clean the skin, then dry the area and apply the creams.

You may also find that using an oil-free moisturizer before putting on the make-up makes it even easier to apply.

Applying with the fingers

If you apply your make-up with the fingers, try doing so with a dabbing motion rather than rubbing, as this will produce a better result. Many people find that they do not get the same level of coverage if they rub the cream on. You may find that you get small bubbles as you dab, but these can be easily smoothed over to create a better finish.

Feather the edges of the made-up area to gradually blend it with the rest of the skin, so that you avoid having a tell-tale clear line between the made-up and unmade-up areas.

Gender comes into it as women might well apply a 'normal foundation' to the whole face prior to applying the camouflage bit and this make blending even easier. Men are likely to want to just cover up the birthmark so need to take a bit more care with the blending aspect of camouflage application and a five o'clock shadow can make this a bit of a challenge!

Hair

In most cases, your make-up will meet your hair at some point. You will probably already be using your hair to cover part of your mark, in which case blending into the hairline will be a little easier.

When you are applying the camouflage cream, it is a good idea to use hair grips to keep your hair out of the way.

For men, there is the questions of when to shave – before or after applying? People do both, but some claim that they get a better result if they apply and then shave. I find that shaving after applying does work, but it does clog up my electric shaver. It is best to experiment and see what works best for you.

Get a mirror

You need a good-quality mirror and good lighting so you can see exactly what you are doing. The quality and intensity of the lighting can make a big difference to how good the make-up looks after you have applied it.

Speaking from personal experience, initially I used an ordinary make-up mirror and a desk lamp, but then I bought an illuminated mirror. It has proved to be an excellent buy as it has made a big difference to the quality of my daily camouflage.

It has three light settings, for 'daylight', 'evening' and 'office', and I am sure now that the desk lamp was giving me a false impression.

If you do use a desk or other lamp, it is a good idea to fit daylight bulbs, which are now available from most outlets. They are blue in colour, but give out a much more natural light than normal bulbs, which enables you to see things more clearly.

Mix it

As noted earlier, some people find that there is a great advantage to mixing two colours to achieve the desired shade. That way you can alter the mix to match your skin tone as it changes due to a suntan and so on. It does take a little longer, so others prefer to stick to one shade, as long as they have been lucky enough to find a good match with a ready-made colour.

If you do mix your own, it is a good idea to try it out a little bit on the skin to see how well it blends in. You can then adjust it by adding a little more of one shade or the other if the test patch does not look quite right.

Variation

Once you have the correct base colour mix, you might want to add a little variation, making the area a bit darker here and a little redder there, for example. This will help it to match the variations that your skin naturally has. If your mark is on one side of your face, look at the opposite side and examine what the skin really looks like. You will probably not want to go as far as Bridget Crawshaw did before her laser surgery, wearing thick camouflage make-up and spending hours dotting on freckles, but, if you feel that you need a better finish, you can improve your technique by creating a slightly less even, more natural effect in this way.

Many women also use blusher to balance out skin colour. For everyday use, you may prefer a matt blusher that does not make the skin glittery.

All over?

Should you use the cream just on the affected area or all over your face? The Red Cross is quite clear on its website that, 'The creams used are not make-up and are used to conceal only the blemish', but one manufacturer says that, as an alternative to covering only the affected area, its creams can be used as an all-over foundation.

Which option you decide on has to be a matter of personal choice and will be affected by the extent of your mark. Some people prefer the all-over method, particularly those with larger facial birthmarks and, perhaps, especially women, for whom the concept of an all-over foundation is not unusual. One advantage is that less colour blending and feathering of the edges are required. You can just put it on and not worry too much about hiding the edges and matching the colour of the rest of your face.

If you do go for the all-over approach, however, bear in mind that you will use a lot more of the expensive creams and, even on prescription, the costs can mount up.

Órla takes the all-over approach, combining general make-up with the camouflage. She uses the camouflage in conjunction with a normal foundation that matches well in colour. You may have to use a slightly heavier foundation than usual to ensure that the camouflaged area does not stand out, but a very good effect can be achieved.

Fixing powder

All the creams require some kind of fixing powder to be applied and this is a very important part of the process. It is a bit like when people appear on television and they have not had sufficient powder applied – they tend to look overly shiny. That is one thing that the fixing powder does – it takes away the unskinlike sheen of the make-up. The other important job it does is to fix the make-up by completing its waterproofing, making it as smudgeproof as possible.

Some powders are translucent, so they can be used over any shade without changing the colour, while others are offered in a number of shades to match different creams. All have instructions for use that vary slightly, but the basic approach is to apply it, leave it for a few moments and then brush any excess off.

Another application trick is to use a damp sponge wrapped in a tissue to remove even the fine bits of powder residue. It also renders the make-up, camouflage or not, more waterproof.

When I first started using the creams and powder, I was amazed to discover just how resilient the finished job is. I can shower, go swimming, work out, even shave, and it still looks fine; it really is waterproof. If you sweat, however, you will notice how the sweat sits differently on the made-up area. It tends to just sit there, which can be a problem as the only way to remove it is to dab it off and with any dabbing or rubbing there is a risk of smearing and smudging. You just need to take a little care with it at such times. If you are at home or can go somewhere private, you could apply a little more powder to absorb the moisture. Many find that the odd dab of powder, just any old pressed powder in a compact, during the day can be a lifesaver – it does not even have to be good-quality.

Sunblock

You should check with the manufacturer as to the sunblock qualities of your camouflage cream and how to use it in conjunction with other sunblock products if required.

Some camouflage products act as a total sunblock as they contains titanium dioxide, the best reflectant available. Properly applied, it blocks *all* harmful rays from the sun, making it more effective than suncreams with the highest SPFs available. Remember, though, that this is not true of all make-up, so, once you have your coverage products and routine, do a little research to check what the situation is for the products you are using to make sure your skin is protected.

Cuts and lesions

The advice here is simple: never use camouflage creams on open skin lesions or unhealed scar tissue.

Removing your make-up

As camouflage creams are made of such wonderfully tenacious stuff, you do need specialist removers to take them off – soap and water will not work.

Ordinary make-up removers and cotton wool will do the job very well or even wipes that have been specially created for removing make-up. There are many brands, but I have found that the cheapest are the supermarkets' own brand versions and they still do a good job.

Órla says, 'Baby oil is an absolute gem, followed by a facial cleanser. Anything oil-based will have your make-up away in a moment – I have even been known to use butter to take my make-up off when I arrived at a hotel without my supplies!'

Ask for large quantities

Check what sizes of container the product is available in and ask for the best-value pot. This will not only save you money, even if you are prescribed it, but it is also good for the NHS as it will also be buying it at the best value. If you only use a small amount of one of your colours, you might choose to get a smaller pot of it so that you can refresh your supply a little more often.

Camouflage creams and fixing powders are non-standard items that pharmacists do not stock as a matter of course, so they have to be ordered in. This can take a week or two in my experience, so try to make sure that you reorder in good time.

Be confident

I have devoted the whole of Chapter 6 to this subject as it really is the key to carrying off the illusion of normal skin that camouflage gives you. All I will say here is that, once you have put it on, forget it and go about your life with renewed confidence.

5

Laser treatment

As mentioned earlier, lasers are used extensively in the treatment of birthmarks. This form of treatment offers a permanent, though sometimes partial, solution, but is not effective for all conditions. Generally, laser treatment is most effective if it is used early in childhood, before the birthmark has thickened and darkened.

Several sessions will usually be necessary, with gaps in between. The number and regularity of these sessions varies from case to case and with the type of equipment, but might number four to six at intervals of four months or up to ten treatments or more at intervals of eight weeks or so. The procedure can be uncomfortable so a local or general anaesthetic may be used, but sometimes none is needed.

Each case is different and will need to be discussed with your consultant. Laser treatments will not necessarily completely remove a birthmark, but they will certainly make it much paler.

How does it work?

The word 'laser' is actually an acronym, the letters standing for 'light amplification by stimulated emission of radiation'. You might be wiser for reading this or you might not! The important point is that laser light takes the form of a beam and the light in the beam is all of the same colour and wavelength. Whereas ordinary light scatters, laser light waves travel together in a single, focused direction. A laser can be 'tuned' to produce light of specific wavelengths, which means that it can be configured to affect only particular colours and densities. You may have seen a famous experiment in which a laser was used to burst a balloon of a particular colour inside a clear balloon. The carefully tailored light was able to burst only the balloon that was the colour it was tuned to, leaving the clear one unaffected.

A medical laser acting on a birthmark is, similarly, tuned to affect only the darker blood vessels within the skin, not the surface. It emits light that will only be absorbed by the red pigment in the blood vessels. The energy of the laser is converted into heat in the skin, which seals the blood vessels that cause a vascular mark, but does not damage the surrounding skin.

There are different types of laser, some gentler than others, and this fact, together with new advances, means that it is worth checking with your consultant about the equipment that will be used, the potential outcomes and any side-effects, such as blistering.

Studies published in the United States suggest that laser treatment is between 40 and 100 per cent effective in removing port wine stains (Roy Geronemus, MD, 'Recommendations for port wine stain treatment', Birthmarks. com, available online at <www.birthmarks.com/HTMLArticle .cfm?Article=272>). It should be remembered though, that this means these marks are, at worst, 40 per cent less visible as a result of the treatment, not that up to 60 per cent of treatments are ineffective. So, these treatments are always effective to some extent and, thus, can make a big difference to people's lives.

Laser treatment for tattoos

As with treatment for birthmarks, pulses of laser light are directed into the tattooed skin. The light passes harmlessly through the top layer of the skin, but is absorbed by the pigment particles in the tattoo. The particles heat up and are shattered into smaller pieces, which can be removed by the body's immune system.

This treatment is usually simple and carries a low risk, but the laser may cause some scarring or pigmentation of the skin. In the latter case, occasionally some of the pigments react with the laser to leave an even darker colour in the skin than was there before. A newer type of laser, used in YAG laser treatment, is particularly good at removing red, blue and black tattoo pigments. However, some colours, such as fluorescent yellow, are very difficult to remove in this way.

Side-effects

There is nearly always some bruising following a treatment session and this can last between 7 and 14 days. The severity will vary. Other than this, the risks are low. As with any wound there is a small chance of infection, which can be treated with antibiotics.

Most port wine stains are treated in around 6 sessions, although this can rise to 12 depending on the size of the stain and how it responds to the laser. The vast majority of improvement occurs after the first three treatments. The face responds best to the laser treatment, limbs less so. Indeed, only 20 per cent of those with stains on their legs can expect good results from laser treatment. As with the face, treatment for marks on the limbs does leave bruising in the area for around ten days afterwards and there is a small risk of scarring

Aftercare

You will need to treat the affected area with care and it is recommended that you avoid products that dry the skin, such as soap, bubble bath and shower gel. Swimming in a chlorinated pool should be avoided at this time for the same reason. You should ensure that you use sunscreen after treatment to protect the skin and prevent discoloration. Your consultant will offer the best advice about aftercare in your case.

The Great Ormond Street Hospital for Children has produced an excellent factsheet with good advice for parents – 'After your child has had skin laser treatment' – which can be downloaded in PDF format (www.ich.ucl.ac.uk/factsheets/families/F020220/after_skin_laser.pdf). There is also a good book for children en-titled *Puss Puss and the Magic Laser* (Pod Publications, 1993: see Chapter 7 in this book for more details).

Information about some other good books can be found by visiting the Skinlaser Directory's website, where you will also find lots of information about laser treatment (<www.skinlaserdirectory.org.uk> – for the books page, click on 'Site map', then 'Publications').

For a photo story for children about laser treatment, visit <www.birthmarks.com> and, once on the home page, click on 'Elizabeth's story' in the box headed 'Our stories', top right, to be taken to 'Goodbye Mr Birthmark' – a story told in pictures. Also in the 'Our stories' box, click on 'Michael's Experience' for a detailed diary with photos of laser treatment going back to 1996 and a streaming video.

Birthmarks.com (www.birthmarks.com) has good photo and narrative material for teenagers and adults, too.

Órla

We met Órla Checksfield in the last chapter. Here is her personal story about receiving laser treatment. As you will see, despite having had some ups and downs, she would recommend laser treatment 100 per cent.

> Why would anybody in their right mind subject themselves to being continually thumped by a light that makes them look like black bubble wrap? This is a question I continually ask myself as I'm going in for a laser treatment.

Six years ago, I decided that it was time to take some drastic action with my port wine stain. My mark covers the bottom quarter of my face, half my neck and the upper part of my chest. It isn't an illness, it won't make me sick in the future, but it does get rather tiring waking up in the morning and seeing a two-tone face looking out at me from the mirror. It is also a pain to wear make-up every day and I know I could go alfresco, but it just isn't me. I've worn make-up since I was two years old, so going out without it now is like going out without a skirt! I also struggle to coordinate my clothes when I'm not wearing make-up. Apparently, this is my own fault because I like to wear pinks and reds and I have been reliably informed by one of my friends that port wine stains do not go well with these colours! She is an expert in this area as she too has a facial port wine stain.

I had tried laser 18 years ago. It was not a pleasant experience, not least because no water was allowed near the treated area for two weeks after the treatment, which led to very greasy hair in my case, but I had heard great things about the pulsed dye laser and I was willing to give it a try.

I went through the normal process of visiting my GP, getting my referral, being assessed, having a patch test (absolutely vital, in order to know what you should expect) and then along came the first full treatment. A full treatment for me is 1200+ zaps. Remember, my port wine stain is rather large – the largest they treat at my hospital in fact. A port wine stain the size of a 50p would probably be more like 15 zaps. In case you hadn't guessed already, 'zapping' is the affectionate term I use for my trips to the hospital every eight weeks or so.

So, off I trotted to hospital. The first step is to put on a topical anaesthetic called EMLA – a cream like a moisturizer that is applied to the area to be treated. Then this is covered in cling film and left to sit for 90 minutes. There is another one called AMETOP that takes effect after 30 minutes, but I am allergic to that one. After 90 minutes, the attractive combination of cling film and cream, which is now a bit more like slime, is removed and I am numb and ready for zapping.

The laser itself is quite a temperamental machine, which must only be addressed with great respect or it breaks down! I once called it a 'bloody thing' on one of my trips and that was it. Another day, one of the nurses addressed it in less than favourable terms and it decided to punish all of those who witnessed this insult by, again, refusing to work. When we all treat the laser nicely, it works, without question. I have been having treatments now for six years and only twice has it refused to play.

The treatment itself has been described in many ways. I think the most accurate description is the following. It is like being hit continually with an elastic band. Now, imagine having an elastic band hit you ten times in a small area and you will understand what it is like to be treated with a laser. Because of this it is also a cumulative pain. The first three zaps are a shock to the system, then you adjust to it and it is OK, apart from some of the sensitive areas – in my case, around my lip area and where my shoulder joins my neck – but, by the time you get to zap 999, your resistance is shot, the anaesthetic isn't quite what it was and it isn't nice after that. Don't get me wrong, it isn't unbearable and I don't whimper my way through the treatment, but it isn't something I would volunteer to do if I didn't know that at the end of it all my port wine stain could be up to 75 per cent lighter.

I come home from the hospital 'nicely bruised'. The hospital likes to see it bruise well because it means that the laser is still having an effect. Let me define 'nicely bruised'. I have described my mark, post treatment, as black bubble wrap and this is definitely the most accurate description I could give. The 'dots' or 'zaps', depending on the settings used, are about the size of the eraser end of a pencil. They are put as close together as the laser operator can manage. The treated dots turn black. See, black bubble wrap. They stay swollen for about 36 hours and then start to subside. The skin stays very red for about two weeks after a treatment, so, until then, I don't know whether I'm happy with the outcome or not.

The treated area must be smeared in moisturizer for about five days after the treatment, as often as I can. In my case, I use petroleum jelly in a 50:50 mix (available from the hospital pharmacy), which is nice and soft. The petroleum jelly, I find, is the only one that doesn't cause the treated area to sting. Scent-free or not, sensitive skin or not, all other moisturizers sting! Everybody mentions ice packs, but I have never been able to get on board with this. No, I am not putting ice straight on my skin. I think it is the severe contrast of the hot skin and the ice pack, even when wrapped in a nice clean, soft cloth, that just doesn't work for me. The skin does feel a bit like sunburn after a treatment and everybody knows what sunburn feels like. A cool cream on sunburn is good, but lumping an ice pack on it may not be as pleasurable.

You also are told not to take painkillers, drink alcohol or basically do anything that will thin the blood and increase the bruising (laser bruising = good; bruising acquired after the treatment = bad, apparently). To be honest, I don't really need the painkillers, but the odd drink would be nice! I guess the upside is at least I can wash my hair from the first day. There are no water restrictions with the pulsed dye laser.

Once the redness has subsided, I can see what has gone on. This can be a tricky time … there are two potential outcomes. I have stared at my port wine stain so often that I cannot see the difference at all or I actually exaggerate the results because I am biased. The reality is my port wine stain has become lighter in colour. How much lighter? Well, one measure I use is to pull out my 'before' photos and then I can easily see the difference. The other is that I used to get through a 20-g pot of camouflage make-up about every three weeks; now they last about eight weeks because I use so much less. My mark is also shrinking in area as the outer edges, which were lighter in the first place, have basically disappeared. Laser treatment is not meant to get rid of 100 per cent of my mark, but it certainly has got rid of a lot of the colour. I can look in the mirror now and notice the black bags under my eyes *before* I see my mark – not necessarily a good thing.

The obvious final question is, 'Would I recommend laser treatment to a friend?' Absolutely! It has certainly been a great result for me. My only stipulation is that you have to want it because, after dot 999 and when the anaesthetic has worn off, all you have is hope and determination.

Remember that Órla has a large mark. You may need fewer than her 1,200 dots, so should not be put off from seeing a consultant if you feel that your determination might not match hers.

Mike

Finally, here is a reminder of what Mike, who we met in Chapter 3, has to say about laser treatment.

My birthmark isn't very big and, coincidentally, looks like a black eye, or so strangers often remark. I've had about seven or eight laser treatments now and it has faded considerably. My doc says 50 per cent, but that was before the last two zaps. I'm pleased with that. It's lighter, smoother-looking and generally softer in appearance.

6
Confidence

You have decided to love your mark and face the world with it or you are about to go out for the first time after laser treatment or wearing your new camouflage make-up. Alternatively, it could be that you are meeting people for the first time or running an event or speaking at a meeting. Whatever challenges you face, being confident will help you to achieve your goals and there is no doubt that, one way or another, those with facial marks have need of a confident approach to help them face the world.

In *The Confidence Book* (Sheldon Press, 2007), I say this about my approach to confidence and it is appropriate here:

> Confidence is not about feelings as we so often think … So this book takes a different approach. We will not try to become more confident people, to change the way we are, the way we feel; rather, we will go at it from the other end and focus on achievement. So the question is not, 'How can I feel more confident in order to make that phone call I've been dreading?'; it is 'How can I prepare to make that phone call to give myself the best chance of success?' If you attack things this way round you'll find that the feelings get dragged along by the action. It's like so many things: focus on the feelings and they become dominant, take action and the feelings can no longer rule.

So, I take a pragmatic approach. Ask yourself what you want to achieve and then work out a way to get there. I suggest giving yourself small (sometimes tiny), but achievable goals, focusing on a step-by-step approach.

I have created a website (www.theconfidencesite.co.uk), which has confidence tips and techniques and more extracts from *The Confidence Book*, as well as links to all the websites mentioned in this book. There is also the opportunity to post your own questions and ideas, but, for the best impact, I heartily suggest that you read the book (well I would, wouldn't I).

In case you think that confidence is somehow the property of 'self-help' gurus, some research by Timothy Judge of Florida University suggests that being confident can help you earn up to twice as much as those who are less self-assured (Cathy Keen, 'Positive self-esteem in youth can pay big salary dividends later in life', University of Florida News, 17 May 2007, available online at <http://news.ufl.edu/2007/05/17/self-esteem>). His study concludes that confident young people who grow into confident adults earn £14,000 more by the time they reach their middle years than their less confident classmates. His view is that confidence is 'the fuel to the fire that leads the advantaged ... to do better'. So, read on and see if you can give yourself a similar advantage.

The effects of stress

Stress is something that we can all suffer from and we all find a source of it – 'It's my job/boyfriend/wife ... or birthmark!' In fact, although we often call it stress, what we are actually experiencing is anxiety caused by stress. Stress is the thing that acts on us, whether it is that we have too much to do, an overpowering boss or a feeling of being 'got at'. Our reaction to it is to feel anxious and this is what we experience.

Terminology aside, I want to suggest that, when we feel this anxiety, there is a way to deal with it. It is not easy and does require perseverance, but it can be overcome. We need not be victims of our feelings, whether they are centred on a birthmark, a perceived idea of 'normal' or any other stress that acts on us. This is not to suggest that we should never feel anxious. Anxiety is an important part of our make-up and it is there for a reason. Imagine that you have left the house and cannot remember if you turned the hob off or not after serving the soup you were making. It is good to feel anxious about this. The anxiety acts as a nagging trigger, a feeling that all might not be well. This turns into a thought: 'I'd better phone home and ask Mandy to check it', or else, 'I'll have to be late for Winston and just pop back and check'.

Sometimes people become overly anxious and, even though they know that they turned the hob off, they feel compelled to check it one more time, then maybe one more time again ... An extreme form of this is the increasingly common obsessive compulsive disorder, but note the terminology – it is a *disorder* of the anxiety response; it does not mean that anxiety itself is a bad thing.

Anxiety is a normal part of the life of a healthily functioning person. It comes from the 'fight or flight' instinct – that state of heightened awareness and readiness for action that evolution has equipped us with so that we can deal with danger. However, things have moved on since we lived by our wits in the wild and modern-day jungles pose problems that are rather different from the ones we had to deal with back then, such as avoiding bites and poison, being on the lookout for animals and others that might attack us and seeking sufficient food and water. However much the modern working or family environment might sometimes feel like we are swimming with sharks and avoiding hissing snakes, those instincts to be on the lookout for danger no longer fit the problems we now have to work on. So, if you were feeling anxious in prehistoric times, you would probably soon take some sort of action, like running away or attacking. Such reactions are not that appropriate in an office, classroom or at home. In other words, our anxiety signals and their causes are out of sync in many cases. We are still stressed by events, but modern life no longer makes practical use of those fight or flight instincts, so we remain in a heightened state with no acceptable release for them.

People who are concerned about their appearance, and therefore feel unconfident in certain social and professional situations, can suffer from this kind of anxiety overload. For example, you might feel anxious if you were going to meet a lot of strangers and worry that they will focus on your mark. Such anxiety builds, but it has nowhere to go. Your instinctive response is to choose fight or flight, but neither is appropriate, so you go to meet the strangers. As you do, you are suitably geared up by your biology to face a perceived threat, but you cannot follow through, so the stress on you increases and your anxiety level goes up.

What you can do about it

As I said above, my approach to confidence issues is to focus not on the feelings but on the situation, and find practical ways forward. That does not mean you should simply pretend that you are not feeling these things.

Step 1 is to recognize what is happening to you. Understand that you are feeling anxious and this is natural. You are not 'bad' because you are feeling 'bad'; it does not mean that you are a failure. You are simply facing stress and your reaction is natural – it is controlled by your hormones, your biology; it is something happening to you, not something that you are choosing.

Step 2 is to apply appropriate strategies, as follows.

Do something physical

Your body is telling you to take action, so, if you can, go for a run or a cycle or do some stretching exercises. You can do anything that will help you physically to discharge the fight or flight imperative. I find swimming is perfect, but it is obviously not always possible to do so. Stretching is a good substitute and can be used in many situations.

Do not dwell on your fears

The more you think about what is worrying you, the more this will stress you and increase your feelings of anxiety as that ancient subconscious instinct prepares your body for action.

It can be a revelation to realize that we can have some control over our thoughts. You can do this in a very literal way by talking to yourself in your mind. I explore this further in the tips for parents in Chapter 7, but the essence is to tell yourself, 'I am not going down that route, I'm not going to dwell on that. Instead, I'll think about ...'.

Train yourself to focus on positive things

... and do it in a positive way! It is better to think about what your strengths are and what you can positively contribute to the situation than it is to focus on the negative. It is equally important, however, to do your positive thinking in a positive way. So, instead of thinking, 'I'll make sure that they don't all stare at my birthmark by being a riveting speaker', say to yourself, 'I'm a riveting speaker and will use all my skills to make an impressive speech'.

Why is the second way better? It is because if you think about things that have a negative connotation – 'Don't all stare at my birthmark' – even if you put them in a positive context, you will be reinforcing that negative idea. So, banish any words that carry with them a negative feeling. Doing so will ensure that you do not open the door that lets all such negative thoughts come flooding back.

Another reason the second version is better is that you cannot actually control how other people will react. So, concentrate on what you can do: be impressive; do not pin your hopes on what you expect others to do in response – in this case, stare or not stare.

Recognize that you cannot change other people

Perhaps in a long-term relationship you and a partner can grow together and affect each other and, over time, change one another, but in the context of the anxiety situations we have been exploring a good place to start is with you. You will be wasting energy and thinking time if you say things like, 'If only she would listen better', 'He should stand up to his boss', 'They focus too much on what people look like and their limited ideas about fashion'.

These are 'their' problem and you cannot change 'them'. Instead, put your energies into what you can change: your attitudes and responses; your strategies and skills for getting your message across.

With this approach in mind, the rest of this chapter is given over to the sorts of confidence issues and questions that people with facial marks raise, with some tips and advice on how to act confidently in a way that will make a difference.

Some common issues

I dread meeting new people because I know that they're only looking at my mark

How do you know that? What gives you that impression?

Can I suggest that you are only assuming they are looking at your mark; you do not know for certain they are. I think it is reasonable to assume that they will look at your mark, but it could be possible that you are exaggerating what has happened. It is simply not true to say that they are *only* looking at your mark. In fact, they may very quickly turn their thoughts away from you altogether.

Given the above, the first step is to gain some perspective. Think this through and tell yourself something like:

- 'They will notice my mark, but they will not be nearly as interested in it as I am. They will quickly normalize my mark, accepting it as just a part of me once it is no longer novel or unusual for them.'
- 'It might take them a little longer to focus on what I have to offer than it would if I didn't have a facial mark, but that's

a small thing and I can easily overcome it or turn it to my advantage.'

Also, do not forget the advice given above – move your thinking away from anything with negative connotations for you and towards what you can offer in a positive fashion. Once you have understood what you are thinking concerning how people might react to you, move on to thoughts about everyday conversations, such as work, sport, a new film.

How can I turn people's reactions to my advantage?

When you first meet someone, walk into an interview or stand up to present, people may well take a moment or two to adjust to the unexpected – your mark. You can use this to your advantage. They were not expecting what they saw, but you were, so plan how to use that temporary uncertainty or disorientation by making an exciting or powerful opening gambit that will quickly bring their attention back to what you are there for. For example, in a presentation, start with a bold, 'Look at this' as you show an inspiring or surprising or even shocking slide. Alternatively, use a powerful quote delivered in a strong, clear manner or play some music that has impact. You have an opportunity to dazzle your audience and seize control of the moment.

If you are meeting someone for the first time, have your opening line ready. This might be as simple as fixing them with a clear but friendly gaze, offering your hand and saying, 'I'm Phil, so very pleased to meet you'. Turn the person's attention from your mark to you. Be direct and you will hold people's attention.

I find it difficult to look people in the eye

Then don't! Look at their eyebrows instead. It will appear the same to them and be easier for you.

My mark is the 'elephant in the room' and I know people want to talk about it

There are a number of approaches to this. The first is, as above, to ask yourself how you 'know' this. It is far more likely to be on your mind and not on other people's. Most might be mildly curious, but not completely fascinated.

If people want to talk about it, that is their decision, not yours. Most people will not ask because they feel uncomfortable about doing so. It is not your job to deal with their discomfort, so leave it to them to ask or not.

If you are concerned about being asked something that you do not wish to respond to, have your answer ready, such as, 'Thanks for asking, but I don't think it's relevant. Have you seen …'.

If, on the other hand, it is you who wants to talk about this elephant, then you need a strategy for how you will do it. You could have a simple factual answer ready, should you be asked, such as, 'No, I don't mind you asking. It's a birthmark, so I've had it all my life. It doesn't hurt at all and it's completely harmless.' I think that it is highly unlikely that you will be asked, however. It has never happened to me among adults. Children are a different matter and quite a few have asked me, 'What is that thing on your face?', 'Does it hurt?', 'Can I touch it?' It is easy to answer these children simply and factually and they quickly move on.

If you genuinely feel that bringing up the subject of your facial mark is important, the best approach is to look for ways to slip it naturally into the conversation, such as:

- 'That reminds me of the last time I had this checked up …'.
- 'Yes, I was bullied a bit as a child because of this mark …'.
- 'It took courage for me to stand up in front of the group that first time, partly because I'm so aware of …'.

Find a support group

There is often quite a drama being played out in our minds – or perhaps it is more of a soap opera or comic strip. However we choose to characterize it, it is very easy to build things up inside our heads and get them out of perspective. Talking to others can make a real difference here, helping you to feel that you are not alone.

You could get in touch with one of the Web-based organizations, such as the Birthmark Support Group and others listed in the Useful addresses section at the back of this book. However you go about it, do not be afraid to talk about your anxieties, practical experiences and the issues that you face. You can do this face to face, on the phone or by email or instant messaging, but I would always recommend that you be cautious about how much you reveal online unless it is with people you know or have at least met. Talking to someone by these methods can be quite seductive and you might be lulled into revealing a great deal of personal information, so always bear in mind the possible dangers.

Many of us are uncomfortable when talking about our feelings, but feelings are real and can be just as powerful and debilitating as physical barriers. I began this chapter by talking about action and a step-by-step approach to change. I therefore recommend that you use your support group to not only get things off your chest but also find practical ways forward.

Talk to someone

If not a support group or in addition to one, find a trusted friend to talk to. We tend to build things up in our heads, imagining more and more dramatic or exaggerated scenarios, so, if you are concerned about something, it is a good idea to talk it through with someone you trust. Get their perspective on the situation and how you come across. Tell them your concerns and listen to their responses. This will help to break the negative mind theatre that may be playing in your head.

There is also the option of finding a professional counsellor or coach to help you, someone who makes it his or her business to listen and help you to reflect and find ways forward. Some people, even in this age of professional help with matters of the mind and motivation, still feel uncomfortable about doing this, but there is really no need to worry. You can hire a personal trainer for your body, so why not do so for your mind and feelings?

Keep trying

By this I do not mean the old adage of 'If at first you don't succeed ...', but, rather, taking the important step of recognizing that the more you put off doing something, the harder it is to do it.

Say you have recently started using camouflage creams and are nervous about presenting the 'new you' to a particular group of people – your family or a group of friends, perhaps. If you leave doing so for a week, you will find that it is harder to take the plunge the following week, even harder the week after that and so on. Try taking it in stages – perhaps arranging to meet one family member or friend first – but do not put it off because you will just be adding to the mental pressure you are putting yourself under by not acting.

Use your positive memories

Often we inhibit ourselves from taking action because we have a mental picture of how it will all go wrong – 'They won't take me seriously', 'I'll be thinking about what they're thinking about my mark!'

Use positive memories from previous experiences to help you. When you find yourself thinking in this negative way, remind yourself that, 'They responded well last time' or 'I was nervous when I started last time, but I soon got over it'.

Extend this by using the technique of visualization. To do this, think yourself back into the positive experience – how it felt after your last successful presentation or when you realized that you had really caught the boss's interest at that interview. Let your mind dwell on the successful event and relive the feelings you had then. You will find that this is an effective way of getting into a positive frame of mind, which will carry over to what you are planning to do.

Order your thoughts

Sometimes our thinking processes can be quite 'leaky'. We might start by feeling nervous about a meeting or event because we feel self-conscious about our facial marks, but, as we think about it, our lack of confidence about that small area then grows until we lack confidence about the task generally.

To combat this tendency, take some time to think about the situation and try to work out exactly what you feel unconfident about and what you can do about it. So, if you feel a lack of confidence because of your facial mark, take a look at some of the ideas in this part of the book and focus on giving the best speech, presentation or whatever it is that you possibly can. Do not allow a general mood of nervousness to develop. Instead, understand why you feel nervous and commit to working on each area individually.

Breathe!

A fairly obvious and automatic thing to do you may think, but it's amazing how taking time to breathe deeply and slowly can make a difference, helping us to calm down and, thus, be more confident.

So, once you realize that you are starting to tense up, for

whatever reason, take a few moments to breathe deeply rather than shallowly from the top of your lungs. Relax, but do not slump, and breathe in slowly through your nose, taking deep breaths from your diaphragm, expanding your stomach until your whole lungs are full of air. Breathe out slowly through your mouth until you have gently emptied your lungs of air. Imagine that, as you breathe in through your nose, you are smelling your favourite flower or food or drink and, as you breathe out, you are causing a candle flame to flicker gently.

Be prepared

The very best way to overcome nervousness is to give yourself as much support as possible. Some people with facial marks, as suggested above, might allow a lack of self-confidence to spread across all their thinking. The solution is to be focused and practical, using the step-by-step approach described above once again.

The following are some tips for giving yourself the best chance of success by planning ahead.

- Work out exactly what you want to get across.
- Decide on your opening couple of sentences and learn them.
- Write down some notes on a sheet of paper or cue cards.
- Rehearse what you will say. Go through it all a couple of times until you feel more confident. Do not overdo this, though – you don't want to appear like a preprogrammed robot!
- Call on the help of a trusted friend or colleague as you do this.

Have a plan

Following on from the above, you might gain confidence from creating a formal plan for whatever you are doing, writing down in advance what you need to say and the key points you want to get across.

This approach can also be of benefit for daily activities, such as putting on your camouflage make-up, if you are new to it. Write down the stages that you need to go through and any tips you might have picked up from others, your own experience or from this book. Work out your routine, write it down, then follow it, perhaps adapting it as you find better ways to do things, until it becomes second nature.

You can adopt a similar approach for meetings with your doctor or dermatologist. Sometimes we are resistant to formalizing things in this way because we think that they are obvious or trivial and we should just be able to do them, but your skin and the face you present to the world are important to you, so why not give yourself the best chance of success, just as you would if you were revising for an exam or following a recipe?

Take the focus off yourself

Following on from the mind theatre that exaggerates the things described above, there are times when we become obsessed with our own issues. Try to monitor your thoughts and feelings so that you become aware when this is happening and have some strategies ready to take you out of yourself. These will vary from person to person, but might include:

- read a book;
- make the effort to meet up with friends;
- phone someone for a chat;
- do some exercise;
- listen to and lose yourself in some music;
- watch an engrossing film;
- write something.

I am a great believer in the value of surfacing things – that is, saying them or writing them down so they become more than vague thoughts or possibilities. So, if you tell yourself, 'The next time I get into that self-obsessed mood, I'm going to break out of it by writing a story or poem or by writing a letter to someone', you will have a better chance of doing so.

Take a walk

Walking is good for us on just about every level. It raises our energy levels, helps to get our creative and thinking juices going and provides healthy exercise.

I do my best thinking when walking. So, if you have something coming up that is causing you anxiety, fit in a walk beforehand if you can.

Take a positivity audit

In everyday terminology, this is counting your blessings and there are plenty of things to be positive about.

If you cannot quite bring yourself to agree to adopt this kind of positive thinking, focus on a great meal you had, your happy or meaningful memories or even a stunning sunset or enjoyable football match. Once you start thinking along these lines, you will see that there is a lot to be genuinely positive about, but you have to make the decision to see the world this way. The alternative is to choose to remain downbeat and concentrate on your problems. I know which I would choose.

Be aware of body language

I once met a teacher with a facial birthmark. It was at a school admissions evening. He had a way of moving his head, as if to shield his mark from people he was speaking to, but, of course, he had a strong imperative to be polite, so he would then turn back again to look people in the eye. Far from shielding and diminishing the impact of his mark, what he was doing had the opposite effect – drawing attention to it as his unusual mannerisms created a sense of unease and the mark was being regularly waved at us.

You can train yourself to become aware of your own body language. Take note of how you sit, stand and move in different situations. Are you performing unconscious actions like that teacher?

Using body language to your advantage

Once we become aware of the effect of body language, we can use it to help us. If you can present a confident picture of yourself, you will feel more confident and so appear more confident. Getting positive reactions will bolster your confidence further, thus creating a virtuous circle.

Think about how you stand. Is your pose a confident one, with your feet firmly planted, slightly apart, giving you a strong, stable image? Try not to rock from foot to foot too much as this is unsettling and suggests that you do not really want to be there. This does not mean that you have to stay rooted to the spot, but neither should you be striding about like Groucho Marx.

If you are sitting, avoid slouching or its opposite – leaning in too avidly, which can be too intense. A comfortable upright seating posture from which you can easily make eye contact (or eyebrow contact – see above) with everyone is the ideal. Look up more than you look down and sweep the room with your eyes (known in training circles as lighthousing), making regular eye contact with your audience (even if it is only two people on the other side of the table).

If you are referring to notes, try to lift them so that your eyes do not keep dipping down towards the floor.

Have a glass of water nearby so that you do not have to worry about a dry throat – this will affect your body language as you become nervous.

Do not be afraid to leave pauses, such as when you take a drink. Your audience will not be going anywhere and not rushing to fill a silence is a sure sign of confidence.

Use your hands for emphasis, but be aware that if you start to wave them around in large movements or too frequently, this will be distracting. You will find that, if you raise them to chest level, your voice will go up too and you will sound more passionate, but also less convincing. How appropriate this is will depend on the situation you are in of course, but as a general rule it is best to keep your hands around midriff level and not overuse them.

You can see that there is a lot to think about with body language, but you should find that, once you begin to think about what you are doing, many things will flow intuitively. A bonus is that, if you are thinking about all this, you will not be worrying about your facial mark!

Write it down

Writing things down is immensely powerful. Most of us allow our thoughts to be rather free flowing, thinking of this, then that, which sparks off a good idea we think we will remember, but then we get distracted and it is all forgotten and so on.

You can use the power of writing things down to help organize your thoughts. So, if you are feeling negative about the effect you think your facial mark is having on your life, give yourself time to write down your thoughts and organize them. It might look something like the example on page 76.

Writing your thoughts down and asking questions of yourself in this way can help you to be more focused and find practical ways forward.

You could also try keeping a regular diary of your experiences, thoughts and feelings. Doing so can help you track your progress and check on past ideas that you may have forgotten

Why I'm fed up

My birthmark is what people notice about me and I'm sick of being 'the one with the birthmark' in people's minds.

Is this true?
I think it's true of Faith and Samina – I saw them looking at me in a funny way – but actually it's not true of all my friends.

So why am I thinking about it?
I guess the truth is that I really would like to be friendlier with Samina. I thought we were going to be great friends when she arrived in the office, but she's disappointed me … No, she hasn't – she probably doesn't even know that I want to be friends.

So what am I going to do?
I'm going to make an effort to talk to Samina at work and maybe invite her along to our team's lunch on Friday. She's only been with us a month, so there's a 'get to know you' excuse …

What about my birthmark?
Actually, it's time that I stopped using it as an excuse. I'm going to investigate camouflage make-up and laser treatment – and there's this great book I saw …

to act on. It is also great therapy to look back on the day as you write and gain some perspective, understanding your emotions and learning from your responses.

Finally

We have met various people in the course of this book, and will meet some more before the end – people with a variety of facial marks and a variety of responses to them, but each has found from somewhere the ability to face the world with confidence. Here are some of the things they say about confidence.

There was one particular incident at a hospital check-up when I was little that is imprinted in my mind. I remember being called in to see the plastic surgeon and when I walked in there he was behind his desk and behind him a row of trainees; it was awful … Now if I've been in a doctor's surgery or wherever and I get asked if I mind students being present I say yes and ask them to leave.

Bridget Crawshaw

Now I realize that most people are perfectly accepting and there is no need to feel paranoid. Many people have 'irrational beliefs' about their scars and marks. However, we are humans and scars and marks are only natural and we should not have to hide them. I threw my make-up away in April 2004 and feel really good about that! Freedom!

Beverley Fulker

Whatever kind of man I am right now and whatever I may grow in spirit to be in the future, my birthmark has helped make me who I am. My life might have been different without it – I may have not been able to see things from the perspective of someone who is unique in a physical way. So I'm glad I have that silly mark. I think it's OK to improve it, just as long as I don't ever forget it.

Mike

I guess I just wanted kids with birthmarks, like me, to have a book with a character they could relate to. I think people who read it will get a better idea of what we [kids with birthmarks] go through every day.

Evan Ducker

Even the earliest, preschool self-portraits of Evan (which I've kept through these last 12 years), include his birthmark. Every drawing, no matter how archaic, bears a red mark on a smiling head, which Evan has always drawn with ease. If there were three stick figures hanging in a row on the classroom wall I could always pick out Evan's! … Just as some kids have freckles and some have dark skin and some are short, Evan has a birthmark.

Donna Ducker

With lots of love and support from my family and friends, and a blossoming self-belief, over the past few years my confidence has grown and grown. I went to university and even fulfilled my dream to become a dancer, before following a successful career in fashion. I now run my own fashion label.

Suzanne Notley

Having a significant birthmark has not stopped me from making friends, enjoying an active social life and forming the normal run of relationships, from girl friendship, boyfriends to permanent partnership ... In the end, I am who I am, not who I might appear to be.

Sarah Earl

7
Advice for parents

In the Introduction, I shared some of my own childhood experiences of having a birthmark and becoming acutely aware of it in adolescence: 'So, at secondary school, my birthmark moved from being a fact to being a factor. It changed from being a thing to being the thing.' Now that I am older, my awareness of and attitudes towards it are different, of course.

I am also a parent and parenthood changes everything. Parents are no longer the centre of their own universes – there is someone else, one or more powerful influences, like planets that have joined our systems, with their own orbits yet part of a new 'us'.

A major factor in all of this is our overpowering desire to protect, look out for, nurture and support our children. It is easy to interpret a perceived threat to them as a declaration of war on you as a parent, an attack on your little universe. So, as parents, we are often ready to react powerfully to threats to our children, which include genuine medical 'threats', such as an illness or injury, and rejection or cruel comments and bullying.

In this chapter, I want to focus on the role that parents and carers can play in supporting children with birthmarks or other facial marks and stress throughout the importance of gaining the proper perspective and understanding because, in all things relating to our children, we owe it to them to offer wise counsel, understand their emotions and equip them as well as we possibly can to face the challenges of life. That sort of thing is easy to say; it is less easy to achieve in the heat of parenting, holding down a job, struggling with your own difficulties and wondering all the time, 'Am I doing this right?' In these situations the tiniest things can push us to the edge, so there is also advice about looking after yourself in order to be the best you can be for your child.

Birth and babies

This is a subject so enormous, so life-changing and powerful that I do not see what I can write to introduce it, so I won't. Instead, I shall let you introduce it yourself. If you have witnessed your child being born or you are waiting for your first child to arrive, either as a mother or partner, you will know how overpowering the emotions, fears, hopes, expectations and experience of parenthood are. I suggest that, somewhere amid the joy, fear and, yes, pain, there will have been anxiety – the thought, 'Is our baby normal?'

'Normal' is a difficult concept, of course, but at this stage you are reassured by the digit count and the healthy cry, the lungs filling with air, but then those other possible concerns appear and one of them will be about your baby's appearance. You take a look and wonder who he or she takes after. You may also notice some kind of mark. As we learned earlier, 1 in 10 children born in the UK has some kind of birthmark. The reassuring thing to know is that 70 per cent of these disappear naturally if left alone. As the parent of a newborn, you will not be able to help but worry and ask yourself what it is and what is the worst scenario.

The good news is that you are in exactly the right place to find out, though perhaps it is not exactly the right time. You are either in a hospital, specialist unit or at home with specialist support staff, so you can ask your midwife, doctor or paediatrician for advice. Be aware, however, that this may not be the best time for you to take in and fully understand what they say to you, so, once you have had a chance to recover from the birth but before you go home or they leave, make sure that you ask again. I wrote elsewhere about my own reluctance to consult my doctor for fear that she would think that I was bothering her with trivial stuff, but, where our children are concerned, especially when they are newborns, we tend to be much more assertive, which is a good thing. You should never feel awkward about asking for advice concerning your child's health. Someone might think that you are being overly fussy, perhaps, but you can live with that a lot better than you could with the feeling that you had let your child down, so be positive and assertive on behalf of your child.

You can also equip yourself with some background information so that you can have an informed discussion. The Internet is a good place to start these days, but, of course, not everything you read will be accurate. Look for the websites of trusted professional organizations, such as the British Association of Dermatologists (BAD). The information leaflets it produces are very good, giving clear information about skin conditions (visit <www.bad.org.uk> or <www.bad.org.uk/patients/leaflets/birthmarks.asp> for details specifically about birthmarks).

One trusted American source of medical advice regarding children is the website of Dr Alan Greene, MD, FAAP (<www.drgreene.com>), who is the paediatric expert for WebMD and the author of several books, including *From First Kicks to First Steps* (McGraw-Hill, 2004) and *Raising Baby Green* (Jossey-Bass, 2007). He is a graduate of Princeton University and the University of California at San Francisco. He teaches medical students and paediatric residents at the Stanford University School of Medicine, which qualifies him as a knowledgeable and well-respected teacher and paediatrician.

You will also find useful advice and information at <www.changingfaces.org.uk>, <www.birthmarks.com> (an American site) and <www.birthmarksupportgroup.org.uk>, but note that none of this, though valuable, should take the place of talking to medical staff about your specific situation. The Web can provide you with a great deal of useful background information, but, like any generalized information, it will not be specific to you or your child. Only a trained professional assessing your child will do where his or her health is concerned.

So, what could this mark be? It could be any one of a number of things – bruising, perhaps, or redness resulting from pressure exerted in the process of being born. The most important thing is that it is unlikely to be serious or life-threatening and it will probably clear up of its own accord over time. You should still ask about it, though, and, if it is still there or seems to be changing over the next few days, ask again. Chapter 1 gives details of the different types of marks there are. To repeat, most do clear up of their own accord, but it is always worth checking things out, as the following story of a child with an unusual type of haemangioma illustrates ('Birthmark nearly blinded daughter', BBC News, 15 January 2006, available online at <http://news.bbc .co.uk/2/hi/uk_news/england/cornwall/4614998.stm>).

Matilda Harding, who lives near St Austell in Cornwall, was born with a birthmark near her right eye that rapidly grew bigger, but her mother was told by doctors it was nothing to worry about and would go away. Three weeks later, the mark had grown and become redder and her eye was swollen and closing up. Then, within weeks, her eye was closed completely and her mother described the mark as being 'like a piece of raw steak stuck to her head'.

Fortunately Mrs Baxter realized that something needed to be done quickly and an Internet search led her to the Birthmark Support Group's website. She sent an email and the BSG put her in touch with Great Ormond Street Hospital for Children. She was seen the next day and an unusual and rapid overgrowth of blood vessels was diagnosed and treated with steroids. Within 12 hours, the mark began to shrink. Without this swift treatment, Matilda's eye might well have been damaged and possibly she could have been blind in that eye.

It should be stressed that cases like this are rare, but it is worth knowing some of the possibilities so that you can have an informed discussion with medical staff.

Positive attitudes to your child's mark

When people say hurtful things

Having a clear medical understanding and diagnosis will help you to prepare for those unfortunate moments when people say hurtful things. Some examples which I discovered in my research include, 'Such a shame for such a pretty baby to have one of those'; 'Can't they do anything about that?' and similar comments.

If you understand the situation, you will be able to say things like, 'It's quite a common birthmark and will probably clear up in a year or so', or, 'It doesn't bother Mahinda or me, so I don't see why it should worry anyone else'.

Keeping a sense of perspective

Be aware of those all too common exaggeration tricks your mind can play on you – 'She's looking at me. I bet she's thinking how odd my baby looks. I wish he didn't look so odd, I wish he was normal …'. That is a typical negative train of thought, set off by what may have been a casual, even admiring, glance. It is so easy to exaggerate things in the theatre of our minds, so guard against it and be aware of times when you do this if you know you are prone to this type of thinking (see Chapter 6 for more details).

Your child has many wonderful qualities that you can celebrate and enjoy. The minor issue of a birthmark, which will probably fade and/or be treated cosmetically, becomes a prominent thing in your mind because of its visual impact. It should not overpower all the wonderful qualities of your baby, a new human being with such potential.

Focus on your child's needs

You cannot do this all the time, to the exclusion of everything else (see below), but, in relation to the comments of other people, put yourself into a frame of mind that enables you to think of your child and his or her needs. What other people think and how they react is their problem; keep your focus on your child and your child's needs alone. If someone says something hurtful, will dwelling on it help your child at all? By all means work through what was said and your own reactions in order to have a better response ready another time, but do not allow it to get in the way of putting your child's needs first.

Talk together

The best advice to give to any couple facing any issue is to talk it through together. Bottling things up inside and not communicating is no way forward in any situation. So, make the effort (and sometimes it can seem like an enormous effort alongside all the other stresses of having a newborn), to talk about it and agree what action you are going to take and how you are going to support each other in practical terms, such as when there are hospital visits and in talks with medical staff. All this assumes that there are two parents involved, but if you are on your own, it is even more important to find someone who will listen and respond, whether this is a parent, sibling or trusted friend.

Sometimes the stresses and anxieties of the new situation we find ourselves in become too much and we find it all but impossible to talk together. In those situations, seek professional help through your health visitor or see your doctor to talk about the possibility of professional counselling. It is not a sign of failure or weakness – you owe it to your baby to look after your own emotional health.

Write things down

If you have a medical visit coming up and are concerned about any aspect of your child's health, write down your questions and any research you have done so that you do not forget what you want to say and can be concise when you have your appointment. It is all too easy in the middle of the topsy-turvy world of being new parents to forget what happened an hour ago, let alone since your last appointment! Keep a notebook with you in which to record your thoughts and questions and go through it before the appointment, pulling out or highlighting the important points.

Looking after yourself

Parenting is hard. It is physically, mentally and emotionally demanding and it can be difficult to find the time and energy for anything else, particularly if you add in concerns about your child's health or appearance. If you do find that you have a moment to yourself, you are likely to want to flop in front of some mind-numbing TV or drift straight off to sleep.

All these things are true, but the effort is worthwhile as it makes such a difference. You will be a better parent if you can feed your own needs as well as those of your baby and other members of the family. If you ignore your own emotional and intellectual needs, as well as your creative and spiritual sides, pretty soon you will become less effective as a parent.

Here are some tips for looking after your own needs in the midst of a busy parenting schedule.

- **Make a plan**
  Give yourself time off on a regular basis by getting a parent, trusted friend or reputable professional to look after your baby and family – perhaps for two hours once a week – and use this time for yourself, in whatever way you choose. You

can spend time together as a couple or by yourself, go out for a meal or to the cinema, whatever is right for you.

- **Snatch any time you can**
  Make the most of any few minutes (they may only be minutes) that come your way to indulge yourself in something that feeds you emotionally and intellectually. Work out what you can do in the odd moments that come your way – arts and crafts, a few pages of a good book, cooking (choose a recipe that you can break off from, though), exercise, even daydreaming.

- **Watch out for negative thoughts**
  As mentioned before, it is very easy when we are tired and drained to allow the negative to take over in our minds. You feel tired, so you feel a bit down, so you think 'down' thoughts – 'This will never end', or, 'I must be a terrible parent'. The trick is to train yourself to become aware of this type of thinking and talk to yourself about it. It is not a sign of madness, it is a very healthy thing to do. You will only be talking in your head, but, if you can say things to yourself such as, 'Yes it wasn't smart to lose my temper, but that doesn't make me a bad parent – I was patient most of the day. I did so many good things for my child today – even a supermum like me is allowed the occasional shout.' Allow yourself to take a step back and see things as they really are, not as your overwrought imagination, fed by tiredness, paints them. (You can find other tips like this for boosting your self-confidence in my book *The Confidence Book* and on its accompanying website at <www.theconfidencesite.co.uk> – you could post a confidence tip there, too, which would be another good way to banish negative thoughts.)

- **Join a support group**
  Find out about any local support groups for parents or even start one of your own for parents of children with birthmarks. Getting the ball rolling can be as simple as putting up a

notice at your local clinic. As with talking with your partner or trusted friend (see above), talking with other parents can be wonderfully freeing and helpful. You tend to think that you are the only one having a hard time or facing a particular problem, but, talking with other parents, you realize that others are going through the same things as you. You can also swap tips and help each other – a little supportive company goes a long way.

Talking with your child about the mark

If your child's mark persists beyond babyhood and into the period where children become vocal and curious about themselves and the world, you will want to think about how to discuss it with them. All parents have to cover difficult or embarrassing topics with their children, whether it is about bodily functions, where babies come from or a whole gamut of other such subjects.

It is best to be honest with children, giving them as much information as they can understand, but also appreciating that their understanding may be different from yours and they may not be able to fully express their feelings or fears. If, for example, they have seen some cartoon or read a book with a laser weapon in it, they might not find it easy to grasp the concept of laser treatment being a good thing however much you explain that it is completely different to the bad guy's laser gun or Zarg's lasermatic destabilizing field. Having said that, children often surprise us with the depth and maturity of their responses to what we might consider to be complicated or awkward situations. Here is an example from the United States.

Evan Ducker was born with a port wine stain on his face. At the age of four, Evan asked his mother why none of the characters in his storybooks had a birthmark. Many children would have listened to their mothers' replies and thought about them, but Evan took things further. His question became the inspiration for a children's book, *Buddy Booby's Birthmark*, which he and his mother created.

Evan loves animals, so he began to dream up a story about Buddy, a booby bird, born with a birthmark. At the time of writing, Evan is 12. Here is what his and his mother's website (www.buddyboobysbirthmark.com) says about the book:

> Journey to the exotic Galapagos Islands, where the native animals just cannot stop talking about Buddy, a newly hatched, red-footed booby bird, born with a birthmark.
>
> Because Buddy is different, he and his mother Isabela, are not exactly welcomed with open arms. However, that does not stop Buddy from being himself and, in the process, teaching the elders some valuable lessons about love, friendship, self-acceptance, and what really matters in life!
>
> When a mysterious Galapagos sea hawk offers to grant Buddy a wish, everyone is sure he will decide to have his birthmark removed. But will he? WOULD YOU?
>
> This imaginative, heart-warming fable has something for everyone.
>
> Kids of all ages will love the rhythm and rhyme of the verses; the bold, expressive illustrations; and learning about the unique creature inhabitants of the Galapagos Islands.
>
> Adults and educators will welcome the timeless messages of self-esteem, tolerance, and the importance of a strong parent/ child bond.

I enjoyed reading Donna and Evan's book – it is an ideal children's story, richly illustrated by Mike Motz and with a simple rhyme structure that even young children will quickly learn so that they will be able join in as you read. The positive message is there, but it's not heavily signposted. The authors allow the story to speak for itself and children will enjoy it on many levels.

We can take a number of inspiring thoughts from Evan's story. One is that working with his mother, who helped him to develop and market the book, Evan was able to make a creative and positive response to his birthmark. He did not see it as a problem, though, I am sure, it created difficulties for him. Evan tells of one experience when, as a young child, he tried to wash off his birthmark. It is interesting to note that he says he did this because 'someone said something and my Mum got real upset', so even then he was not concerned for himself but for his mother and her reaction. Through his book, Evan was able to take his situation and turn it into something life-enhancing, for him and for other children and parents. This is testament not only to Evan's attitude but also to the loving and supportive parenting he received. 'I guess I just wanted kids with birthmarks, like me, to have a book with a character they could relate to,' says Evan. 'I think people who read it will get a better idea of what we [kids with birthmarks] go through every day.'

Evan and his mother have made use of one of the defining abilities of human beings – being creative and using metaphor to help us make sense of and cope with our lives. Children do this all the time in play, trying out 'as if' stories of being parents or superheroes, working through their anxieties and hopes using their imagination, and that is what Evan and his mother have done with their story. It was not enough just to talk about Evan's mark; they found a way of dramatizing it and its effect on Evan and other people and, in so doing, worked out what they thought about it and how to live more positively.

You can do this, too. When the time is right, which is usually when your child raises the issue, build characters with birthmarks into the stories you tell or the pictures your child paints. If he or she creates an image of someone with a mark, gently pick up on this and respond to it. You could even choose a character together from a storybook and draw a birthmark on it. This can send a powerful message because 'Big Ted', for example, is just the same as he always was, doing the same things with a birthmark as he did without it.

There are endless ways in which you can include birthmarks in imaginative activities, which helps to make them normal, just a part of everyday life. These provide opportunities to talk and work through issues and anxieties using the power of imagination.

One more thing you could do is take a look at Evan's book on the website and order one.

Evan's mother, Donna, notes:

> It's funny you should mention the pictures and adding birthmarks because, even the earliest, preschool self-portraits of Evan (which I've kept through these last 12 years), include his birthmark. Every drawing, no matter how archaic, bears a red mark on a smiling head, which Evan has always drawn with ease. If there were three stick figures hanging in a row on the classroom wall I could always pick out Evan's! And, his friends would often draw pictures of themselves with Evan (and he'd have his birthmark). So, it was never a 'bad' thing, it was just a natural part of Evan. Just as some kids have freckles and some have dark skin, and some are short, Evan has a birthmark.
>
> It's such a non-issue to us – *that's* the message we wanted to get out to people with *Buddy Booby's Birthmark*. It's not a defining thing, it's a describing thing. Evan is a great, talented, compassionate, bright, funny kid who has brown hair, brown eyes and a birthmark. Nothing to be ashamed of, nothing to hide with make-up and nothing to do with the kind of friend he is, or the contributions he will make to society, or any of the things that matter. I know that. He knows that. We just wanted the rest of the world to be reminded of it, because it seemed many people had forgotten it somewhere along the way.

In the UK, there are a number of books written by Doreen Trust and illustrated by Peter Trust, published by Pod Publications, available from the Disfigurement Guidance Centre (DGC) and the Skinlaser Directory's website, where other books are also listed (see the Useful addresses section at the back of this book for contact details). The books have charming pictures with fun and often quirkily humorous text. There are also opportunities for children to discuss the stories and their concerns. In some cases, there are pages for the children to complete themselves.

- *Puss Puss and the Magic Laser* (Pod Publications, 1993) tells of a cat that loves colour and rainbows. When she goes to the laser clinic for her birthmark treatment, she is naturally curious about what will happen and how it will all work. The story includes information about aftercare and is immensely helpful to any young child who will be visiting a laser clinic.
- *The Mouse with Pink Ears* (Pod Publications, 1994) is a delightful story told by a mouse who feels self-conscious about its appearance and finds the confidence to move from 'I suppose the first thing you noticed about me were my pink ears ...' to 'I suppose the first thing you noticed about me was that I'm a mouse'. The short text and imaginative illustrations make for a charming book for both adults and children, with a gently delivered message that all children will benefit from.
- *Does the Way You Look Really Matter? How to improve your self-esteem and become a social super-dragon* (Pod Publications, no date) This is a wonderfully quirky book with questions to answer and things to think about, leading to the important message:

LIKE me,
LIKE others,
LIKE life,
GREAT!

It is hard to pin down with regard to age range as children and adults will find fun and helpful information inside. It reads like a very original type of self-help book.
- *About Disfigurement* (Pod Publications, 1995) This is a book for older children, teenagers and adults, but it keeps the fun style of the books aimed at young children. It is described as 'The essential guide to help those who care for men, women and children who are disfigured: What to do as well as what not to do'.

Discuss treatment options

When appropriate, you will want to run through the various treatment options with your child. Again, it is best to be open and honest and the support of others can be crucial. The Birthmark Support Group (BSG) runs a number of fun days at different locations around the UK and these provide a great opportunity for children and parents to get together; an ideal setting for the exchange of information and for you and your child to get first-hand knowledge and support about the various treatments available.

Adolescence

Any parent will have their hands full as their children move from childhood to adolescence or, in fact, their hands will be emptier as they learn to let go! Your child's attitude to his or her mark may well change during this time. Some want to hide it for the first time or have its impact lessened by having laser treatment or using camouflage and others are the opposite, suddenly forgetting about it as other things take over.

Many of the people I have spoken to said that having a birthmark has not prevented them from forming significant relationships, but this was a real concern in their adolescence. They felt inhibited or, in some cases, convinced that they were too ugly to be of interest to potential boyfriends or girlfriends.

All you can do to help your child at this time is all that any parent can do – try your best! Take a deep breath and don't take it personally if your offers of help are dismissed or even angrily rejected. Try to listen to what your child says, but store things away so that you can process them later with the benefit of being in a calm state and ask yourself, 'What was that *really* about, what is my child really saying here, what practical help can I offer?' Also, remember that all adolescents have to find some focus for their angst and, in a strange way, your child's birthmark might seem more normal amid the eruptions of pimples around your child at school and in their peer group.

Once again, talking with other parents will help so do take full advantage of the support groups available.

There is an excellent factsheet available from Great Ormond Street Hospital for Children: 'Bringing up a child whose face looks different' (available online at <www.openspace.nhs.uk/factsheets/families/F010115/index2.html> and, for other general information, visit the home page at <www.ich.ucl.ac.uk>).

Parent and child activities

I wrote above about how helpful reading and drawing together can be when talking with your child about his or her birthmark. Here are some more activities that parents or carers and children can do together to help bring concerns out so you can discuss them and build confidence.

'People we like' collage

Make a collage together using pictures from magazines. Discuss the images you see and why you chose to use them. Some might be famous people who are known to your child, others might look fun to be with or have a kind face.

The aim of this activity it to try to get across the idea of diversity and the value of being different, of how dull the world would be if everyone looked the same. You could include some pictures of people with birthmarks (see the various Internet sites mentioned in this book for material).

Do not forget to include your child, yourself and your family!

Doll treatment

If your child is undergoing laser treatment or beginning to use camouflage cream, you could draw a mark on a doll using felt-tips and then cover it up or clean it off as your child's treatment progresses. Alternatively, you can do this in advance of treatment as a way of talking about and showing what will happen in the sessions.

If you are handy with a needle and thread, you could make a birthmark for a fabric doll, although it would be harder to change it to match the improvements as treatment progresses.

You could take either doll to your medical appointments and ask the consultant to show your child what will happen using the doll. This can help a child to understand more clearly what the treatment will involve.

Board game

Make a board game together that addresses any concerns your child has, whether they are about feeling different, being picked on, medical treatment or general confidence issues.

The game need not be elaborate – the fact that you have made it together will make it much more playable than something from a shop and, besides, the making is the most important part, as you talk together about these issues and what will be on the squares and any cards that players pick up. Here are some examples to get you started.

- Go to see special doctor. Go forward three squares.
- Have a great time playing with Mum's make-up. Go forward one square.
- A silly person tries to hurt your feelings, but you are kind back. Go forward five squares.

More books

I mentioned *Buddy Booby's Birthmark* above, which is specially written for children with birthmarks, and some other books from Pod Publications, but there are plenty of other children's books that also touch on issues of confidence, being yourself and not worrying about what others think. For younger children, many books from specialist children's publishers such as Barefoot Books (www.barefoot-books.com) can be used to discuss issues of bravery and confidence. Here are some that you may like to take a look at.

- Jen Wojtowicz, *The Boy Who Grew Flowers* (Barefoot Books, 2005) A delightful modern fairytale.
- Jules Bass, *Herb, the Vegetarian Dragon* (Barefoot Books, 2005) Teaches us that it is all right to be different, even if you are a dragon.
- Tanya Batt, *The Faery's Gift* (Barefoot Books, 2005) A humble woodcutter learns to trust himself.
- Hugh Lupton, *The Story Tree* (Barefoot Books, 2005) Includes confidence-building tales for young children.

For older children, the notion of being the one special person who has to cope against the odds is a staple storyline, Harry Potter being a classic example. You can use this idea to give your child confidence when he or she has to face a difficult or uncomfortable situation.

You can find one of my own stories for younger children, *The Sound the Hare Heard*, on The Confidence Site (<www .theconfidencesite.co.uk>). It is based on a Buddhist fable and is about being confident to be yourself, not simply following the herd. There are no illustrations so, as another activity, you could illustrate the story with your child, creating your own book. You do not have to copy out all the words – just tell the story in pictures. If you do want to include some of the text, you can download the story from The Confidence Site, print it off and cut it up or, if your child is a computer whizz, he or she could copy and paste, doing the whole thing electronically. I hope you find it useful and that it leads to some interesting discussions.

Two inspiring stories

To end this chapter, here are two stories that I hope will inspire parents who may be worried about what their children will have to deal with because they have facial marks.

The first is the story of Suzanne Notley, in her own words (you can see Suzanne tell her story on video at <www.bbc.co.uk/ cambridgeshire/videonation/content/face_value.shtml>). She reminds us of the very real, though thankfully rare, dangers of some types of birthmark, but goes on to offer key messages about the support of parents, the importance of support organizations and, crucially, of self-belief and motivation.

Hi there, I'm Suzanne, I'm 30 and live in Wisbech, Cambridgeshire (England, UK). About a week after I was born, an outline appeared on my face around my right eye. This developed into a strawberry haemangioma, which grew and became very heavy, sealing my eye shut. As the mark was over my eye and there was a risk of losing my sight, I had an operation to remove some of the birthmark, but, unfortunately, my sight could not be saved and I cannot see out of my right eye at all. I then had two further operations to 'tidy up' the quarter of my face that was affected by the mark. Like many of us, I suffered times of low self-esteem – during my teens I wore my hair over my face and even refused to put make-up on my 'bad eye', thinking that if I ignored it everyone else would as well! I also have further birthmarks down the right side of my body, from my bottom to my toes, which made PE and swimming at school a real misery. I did try camouflage make-up and laser treatment, but soon gave up – it just wasn't for me.

With lots of love and support from my family and friends, and a blossoming self-belief, over the past few years my confidence has grown and grown. I went to university and even fulfilled my dream to become a dancer, before following a successful career in fashion. I now run my own fashion label, Fashion Junkie, for women sized 10 to 32, alongside being mummy to baby Olivia Grace. I used to be so nervous of being photographed, but have now appeared in various articles in national newspapers and magazines about my birthmarks – talking about it all has been such a liberating experience and I hope that reading about me has helped others, too. I wish that Birthmarks.com and the Birthmark Support Group (UK) had been around when I was a child. Having people with similar experiences to talk to would really have helped my parents and me in so many ways.

To end, here is Sarah Earl's story, which she tells in her own words.

I can't remember a time when we, as a family, didn't talk about my birthmark. I was never made to feel ashamed of what was merely an accident of birth.

As a child, I was aware of being 'different' – people would stare in the street, children in queues would ask their parent(s), or sometimes me directly, 'What is wrong with your face?' I was always encouraged to explain, even though the parent(s) often displayed embarrassment – I felt I needed to put them at their ease!

The people who stared at me in the street often made me feel angry, but Mum would stare down the most blatant starers and, eventually, I started doing the same. This was not out of malice, but helped to empower me, because both Mum and I are aware of looking at the 'different' ourselves. As I grew older and we discussed it as a family, I became aware that some people stare out of curiosity, some out of embarrassment and a few out of ignorance. It also is important to be aware that we as human beings are programmed genetically to quickly identify and eliminate as a threat anyone whose facial characteristics do not conform to the norm. This knowledge helps me to come to terms with other people's responses. It's natural to suspect this response of being malicious, although in reality this is very rare.

I was lucky to have a supportive, loving and intelligent family who were always prepared to discuss these issues and who were always very supportive and positive. I was frequently told that not only was I beautiful, but the people who would matter to me would only ever see my birthmark once and happily this has proven to be the case.

As a young girl, the first boy who asked me out on a date was a tremendous confidence booster.

This is not to say that I haven't been the brunt of the negative side of human nature. I've experienced the usual name-calling and bullying, which were traumatic and hurtful.

I went through a phase of trying to cover up or eradicate the birthmark via make-up, which I hated, and laser treatment, which was fairly effective but unpleasant, and, although not a consideration on their part, it was expensive for my parents. I reached a point where I simply felt enough was enough and people could take me as I was or not – it would no longer be my concern. This philosophy has stood me in good stead to this day.

Having a significant birthmark has not stopped me from making friends, enjoying an active social life and forming the normal run of relationships, from girl friendship, boyfriends to permanent partnership. My mum is a great believer in 'nature' rather than 'nurture', but, without the positive attitude of my family, maybe I wouldn't feel as confident as I do today, who knows?

In the end, I am who I am, not who I might appear to be.

Useful addresses

You can find an electronic version of these pages at The Confidence Site, <www.theconfidencesite.co.uk>, which gives easy access to all the links below.

NHS-based resources

For many UK readers, the NHS will be the first port of call for information. There are two major NHS sources to recommend – NHS Direct and the Skin Disorders Specialist Library.

NHS Direct
24-hour helpline: 0845 4647
Website: www.nhsdirect.nhs.uk

NHS Direct is accessible via either telephone or a large website that covers a vast range of conditions and possible treatments. The easiest ways to navigate it are to use either the fast and efficient search option, typing in a word or words in the search box, or the 'Health encyclopaedia' and search using the A–Z index.

Skin Disorders Specialist Library
Website: www.library.nhs.uk/skin/

Note that this is described as being mainly for specialists: 'Patients, carers and the general public are welcome to use this site, but may wish to visit NHS Direct Online first'. So, you can find out some background information, but some of the detailed information is quite advanced.

General

Barefoot Books
124 Walcot Street
Bath BA1 5BG
Tel.: 01225 322400
Fax: 01225 322499
Email: info@barefootbooks.co.uk
Website: www.barefoot-books.com

The children's books mentioned in the book published by Barefoot Books can be found on its website. You can choose to visit the UK or US version and then search for the title you are interested in.

The Birthmark Support Group
London WC1N 3XX
Tel.: 0845 045 4700
Website: www.birthmarksupportgroup.org.uk

A UK-based charity whose patron is Esther Rantzen, the group was set up
by parents of children with birthmarks in December 1998 at the suggestion
of doctors from Great Ormond Street Hospital. Its objective is to provide
a UK-based support group for anyone with a birthmark, and now covers
both children and adults. It is a friendly organization run by people who
understand the issues from the inside, and has a good deal of useful
information and networking opportunities on its website, including details
of its 'Fun Days'.

British Association of Dermatologists
Willan House
4 Fitzroy Square
London W1T 5HQ
Tel.: 020 7383 0266
Website: www.bad.org.uk
Email: admin@bad.org.uk

The BAD is the central and long-established association of practising UK
dermatologists, the aim of which is to continually improve the treatment
and understanding of skin disease. Its website is provided as a resource for
members of the public searching for reliable information about the skin
and skin diseases. You will find an excellent selection of leaflets in PDF
format, including information on birthmarks.

British Association of Skin Camouflage
PO Box 202
Macclesfield SK11 6FP
Tel.: 01625 871129
Website: www.skincamouflage.net/
Email: basc9@hotmail.com

The association provides plenty of details about camouflage products and
their use and publishes a magazine – *The Cover* – that keeps readers up to
date. There is also information about training courses.

British Red Cross
UK Office
44 Moorfields
London EC2Y 9AL
Tel.: 0870 170 7000
Fax: 020 7562 2000
Website: www.redcross.org.uk

This is a well-known UK charity that has His Royal Highness The Prince of Wales as its president. It runs skin camouflage clinics throughout the country, offering advice, colour matching and training. It will also fill in the forms that enable your GP to write prescriptions for the creams you need. Either use the well-designed search function to find references to 'Camouflage', which will bring up a list, then you can find your nearest clinic, or click on 'Your local area' in the 'Quick links' list on the home page and keep choosing options until you are given a list of 'Available services', then choose 'Skin camouflage'. For local offices and shops, you can also enter a postcode in the 'Your area: Find your local services' box on the home page. Alternatively, as you will need your GP to refer you to use the service, he or she should also be able to provide you with details of your nearest clinic.

Changing Faces
The Squire Centre
33–37 University Street
London WC1E 6JN
Tel.: 0845 4500 275
(From outside the UK): 00 44 20 7391 9270
Website: www.changingfaces.org.uk

Changing Faces Cymru
Tel.: 0845 4500 240
Email: cymru@changingfaces.org.uk

Changing Faces Northern Ireland
Tel.: 0845 4500 732
Email: nireland@changingfaces.org.uk

Changing Faces Scotland
Tel.: 0845 4500 640
Email: scotland@changingfaces.org.uk

A charity providing support and information for children and adults who have any form of disfigurement. It aims to help with coping strategies and self-confidence and works with healthcare professionals, schools and others to promote awareness of disfigurement and its effects.

Contact a Family
209–211 City Road
London EC1V 1JN
Tel.: 020 7608 8700 or 0808 808 3555 (helpline: 10 a.m.–4 p.m., Monday to Friday, plus 5.30–7.30 p.m., Monday)
Fax: 020 7608 8701
Email: info@cafamily.org.uk
Website: www.cafamily.org.uk

A UK charity that provides support and advice to parents whatever the medical condition of their child. Enter 'birthmark' in their search box for useful information and to set up contacts.

Great Ormond Street Hospital for Children NHS Trust (GOSH)
Great Ormond Street
London WC1N 3JH
Tel.: 020 7405 9200
Website: www.ich.ucl.ac.uk

GOSH offers a great deal of helpful and accessible information for parents and children, including the fact sheets mentioned in this book. The fact sheets may be accessed through the menu system (Publications>Factsheets) or at this url: <www.gosh.nhs.uk/factsheets>. Information is available also in Arabic, Bengali, Greek and Turkish.

Skinlaser Directory
PO Box 7
Cupar
Fife KY15 4PF
Scotland
Tel.: 01337 870281
Website: www.skinlaserdirectory.org.uk/Publications.htm

This directory provides doctors and patients with essential facts about skin lasers and skin laser treatments. It also provides information about a number of publications, including Pod Publications: books for children.

Sturge Weber Foundation (UK)
Burleigh
348 Pinhoe Road
Exeter
Devon EX4 8AF
Website: www.sturgeweber.org.uk

A UK-based charity offering information and advice on this rare condition.

Websites

www.birthmarks.com

An American website with an excellent range of articles and background information covering laser treatment, camouflage and mentoring, giving advice and personal stories for all ages. The story section is worth spending some time exploring as it contains a wealth of experiences and much wisdom. There is a photo story for children about laser treatment. On the home page, click on 'Elizabeth's story' in the box headed 'Our stories', top right, to be taken to 'Goodbye Mr Birthmark' – a story told in pictures. Also in the 'Our stories' box, click on 'Michael's Experience' for a detailed diary with photos of laser treatment going back to 1996 and a streaming video. Birthmarks.com also publishes an online newsletter, covering a variety of topics relating to birthmarks, including contributions from people living with birthmarks, those outside the community, such as experts of various kinds (dermatologists, make-up artists, psychologists, laser surgeons, specialists, journalists and so on), and Birthmarks.com's sponsors.

The Confidence Site

www.theconfidencesite.co.uk

The website that supports my book *The Confidence Book* (Sheldon Press, 2007) has opportunities to read and post confidence tips and a 'Confident Kids' section.

Dermnetnz.org

http://dermnetz.org

This site, based in New Zealand, has an extensive range of useful information about skin diseases, conditions and treatments.

Disfigurement Guidance Centre

www.timewarp.demon.co.uk

Linked with the International Skinlaser Directory (see above).

Dr Greene

www.drgreene.com

A trusted American web source for medical advice regarding children, the site carries information on a very wide range of childhood conditions, including birthmarks and other facial abnormalities. The site can be contacted through a web form on the 'Contact Us' page.

Let's Face it Support Network
Tel.: 01843 833724
Website: www.letsfaceit.force9.co.uk

A contact and support network site with a newsletter, features and articles. It aims to offer friendship, support and assistance. Its founder, Christine Piff, suffered a facial cancer resulting in the loss of half her face and formed the network as a result of the experience.

Vascular Birthmarks Foundation Europe
http://vbfeurope.org
American site: www.birthmark.org

This site provides lots of detailed information, including a translation service into English, Spanish, French, German, Italian and Portuguese; also a unique 'Ask the Doctor' service using a web-based form which is supported on a volunteer basis by physicians who work with VBF. Note: *You are requested to use this personal service only if you are unable to find the information you need on the extensive website.*

Further reading

Bass, Jules, *Herb, the Vegetarian Dragon*. Barefoot Books, Bath, 2005.

Batt, Tanya, *The Faery's Gift*. Barefoot Books, Bath, 2005.

Ducker, Donna and Ducker, Evan, *Buddy Booby's Birthmark*. Xlibris Corporation, Philadelphia, PA, 2006 (available online at www.buddyboobysbirthmark.com).

Lamont, Gordon, *The Confidence Book*. Sheldon Press, London, 2007.

Lupton, Hugh, *The Story Tree*. Barefoot Books, Bath, 2005.

Trust, Doreen, *About Disfigurement: The essential guide to help those who care for men, women and children who are disfigured: What to do as well as what not to do*. Pod Publications, Cupar, 1995.

Trust, Doreen, *Does the Way You Look Really Matter? How to improve your self-esteem and become a social super-dragon*. Pod Publications, Cupar, [no date].

Trust, Doreen, *The Mouse with Pink Ears*. Pod Publications, Cupar, 1994.

Trust, Doreen, *Puss Puss and the Magic Laser*. Pod Publications, Cupar, 1993.

Wojtowicz, Jen, *The Boy Who Grew Flowers*. Barefoot Books, Bath, 2005.

Index